T0076132

Advance Praise for *Everyday Miracles*

"Propelled by compassion and intellect, Dr. Richard Burt's journey of scientific discovery led to a breakthrough treatment for autoimmune disease resulting in hundreds of sufferers living disease-free. *Everyday Miracles* is his story and theirs—displays of courage and perseverance against conventional thinking and disease will find you in awe on one page and angry on another. As a catastrophic illness survivor, I, along with my family, share the gratitude felt by the individuals profiled in this book and we are very thankful for Richard's brilliant mind and compassionate heart. As a former United States congressman and senator, [I know] there is much to gain from following Dr. Burt's lead and challenging conventional wisdom on the treatment of disease."

—**U.S. Senator Mark Kirk (IL)**

"Dr. Richard Burt tells us in *Everyday Miracles* that 'Medicine is the interface between the humanities and science.' The author's fascinating journey takes us on our own discovery of humanity and medical and healthcare systems and structures for advancing knowledge and healthcare. Dr. Burt has a unique voice and a powerful set of stories to tell."

—**Professor Henry Bienen, PhD, President Emeritus,**
President Northwestern University (1995 to 2009)

"An inspirational book by a pioneering physician whose humanity and empathy shine from every page. Dr. Burt really understands the terrible toll of autoimmune conditions—the pain of gradually losing one's essential self to MS or Crohn's disease—and has dedicated his life to finding a new answer. It's a must-read for patients and doctors alike."

—**Caroline Wyatt, Award-winning International Broadcaster**
and Journalist

"Inspiring and often deeply humanistic. In *Everyday Miracles*, Professor Richard Burt, the preeminent physician-scientist in the field of stem cell transplantation for autoimmune diseases, offers insight through a beautifully written book into a pathway for hope and cures."

—James Mason MD, Professor of Medicine,
Scripps Clinic, USA

"As a physician looking after people with multiple sclerosis, I found this book to be both moving and insightful. Its heartwarming stories give an accurate reflection of the true cost of this devastating illness and the human ingenuity [that's needed] trying to find a cure for it. This is an essential read for everyone with multiple sclerosis, systemic sclerosis, or other autoimmune diseases."

—Basil Sharrack, PhD, Professor of Neurology,
University of Sheffield, UK

"*Everyday Miracles* is an engaging explanation of a new treatment that has fundamentally changed the natural history of multiple sclerosis and other autoimmune diseases. It is out-of-the-box thinking that advances science and medicine with a depth of conscience. Its impact will extend well beyond these diseases and patients as it teaches us about the ethics of our societies and medical care. It is a window into curing diseases and a window into ourselves."

—Dominique Farge MD, PhD, Professor of Medicine,
Université Paris-Cité, France

EVERYDAY MIRACLES

Curing Multiple Sclerosis, Scleroderma, and
Autoimmune Diseases by Hematopoietic Stem Cell Transplant

PROF. RICHARD K. BURT, M.D.

Forefront
BOOKS

Everyday Miracles: Curing Multiple Sclerosis, Scleroderma, and Autoimmune Diseases by Hematopoietic Stem Cell Transplant

Copyright © 2023 by Dr. Richard K. Burt

All rights reserved. No part of this publication may be reproduced, stored in a retrieval system, or transmitted in any form by any means, electronic, mechanical, photocopy, recording, or otherwise, without the prior permission of the publisher, except as provided by USA copyright law.

No patent liability is assumed with respect to the use of the information contained herein. Although every precaution has been taken in the preparation of this book, the publisher and author assume no responsibility for errors or omissions. Neither is any liability assumed for damages resulting from the use of the information contained herein.

This book is intended for informational purposes only. It is not intended to be used for the sole basis for medical or health decisions, nor should it be construed as advice designed to meet the particular needs of an individual's situation.

Published by Forefront Books.
Distributed by Simon & Schuster.

Library of Congress Control Number: 2022914872

Print ISBN: 978-1637631256
E-book ISBN: 978-1637631263

Cover Design by Bruce Gore, Gore Studio, Inc.
Interior Design by PerfecType, Nashville, TN

I wrote this text for patients with autoimmune diseases. There is hope, and with all new advances, new doors open, but new questions and difficulties arise. I want to thank my patients for their trust and strength.

I also thank Shalina, Michael, Rajan, Reena, and Shantha for tolerating my indulgence in opening a new frontier. Their faith and support were extraordinary.

Finally, I want to convey my gratitude to all the positive-energy people, both within and outside the medical field, who supported me on this journey.

CONTENTS

THE DALAI LAMA

FOREWORD

I marvel at the advancements that have been made in science and
technology, particularly developments in stem cell transplantation, where a
person's own cells are used to treat previously incurable ailments. I
therefore welcome this book that details several cases of individuals who
have benefited from such medical developments.

Coincidentally, I came to know two of the individuals mentioned in the book
who were witness to Tibetan demonstrations in Lhasa in 1987 and thereafter
did much to spread awareness of the plight of the Tibetan people.

This book celebrates individual accounts of the human spirit prevailing
despite intense physical suffering and odds. The personal experiences
mentioned also emphasize the importance of the loving support of family
and friends in these stories of triumph over desperation and hopelessness.

I hope the book "Everyday Miracles" by Dr. Richard K. Burt, will be an
inspiration for people to continue looking for ways to benefit from scientific
developments and acts of loving kindness by near and dear members of our
human family.

18 May 2022

CHAPTER 1

ERETRIA VERSUS CRUELLA
HSCT versus Multiple Sclerosis

A few months before her twenty-first birthday, Eretria thought she was losing her mind. When she closed her eyes, she saw daylight—vertical lines waving back and forth with light shining through like a partially drawn shade on a sunny day. She was too scared to tell people for fear they would think she was going crazy.

New symptoms developed while she was taking a shower. Eretria had to put her head and body against the shower wall to keep from falling over. She pushed against the wall to balance herself as she walked around and out of the shower. Her hands shook so hard, it was difficult to dress. She could no longer put on makeup. Her arms and legs became numb. She turned to her grandmother, who had always been there for her.

Eretria's grandmother took her to a doctor, who diagnosed a stroke and sent her home. Eretria was not trained in medicine. She was only twenty-one years old, but at her young age, she felt a stroke could not possibly be correct. Frustrated by her continued symptoms, she went to the emergency room and was hospitalized. After basic lab work and a drug screen, which all came back normal, she was diagnosed as a hypochondriac and discharged.

Eretria knew herself and knew she was not a hypochondriac. She reasoned that either her symptoms were real, or she was truly going insane. Either way, something was seriously wrong. She sought a third opinion at another hospital, and, after a brain imaging (MRI) study, she was diagnosed with multiple sclerosis (MS), a chronic incurable disease in which your body's own immune cells attack your brain and spinal cord. They treated her with steroids and Cytoxan (an immune-specific chemotherapy).

Attacks and hospitalizations occurred so frequently that Eretria ended up on a first-name basis with the hospital staff. Just a year earlier, she had been a carefree twenty-one-year-old girl thinking about makeup, going out with her girlfriends, and dating. She wondered when the next *Cosmopolitan* magazine would arrive in the mail. She never imagined she would soon be reading an MS magazine next to someone in a wheelchair while being infused with steroids herself.

She was placed on disability due to frequent work absences when she was hospitalized for relapses of MS. Eretria's job had given her purpose. The rug was pulled out from under her when she lost it. By her mid-twenties, she had no money, no job, no support. Her grandmother, who had always been by her side, got sick and could not care for her, nor could she care for her grandmother. Due to drug side effects, to get to the bathroom on the nights when she took her MS injections (interferon), she had to crawl across the floor. She would put her hands on the toilet to lift herself up. Eventually, on the nights of her interferon injections, she would just sleep on the bathroom floor.

Medically, things continued to worsen for Eretria. She started using a cane. Her vision declined. To get urine out of her body, she had to intermittently self-catheterize (insert a tube into) her bladder. The money she got from disability was not nearly enough to pay for interferon injections that cost $90,000 a year. To make ends meet financially, she was forced to skip some interferon injections, started going to soup kitchens, and sleeping in cars. She was not a stereotypical street person (if there is any such thing). She was educated, polite, beautiful, thin, appropriately proportioned, and had a dazzling white smile with perfectly smooth skin. She is of Italian descent with dark, piercing, and entrancing eyes.

Eretria is a real-life Cinderella. The only difference is that she was not facing a sadistic stepmother named Lady Tremaine. She faced an enemy even worse than either Disney character Lady Tremaine or Cruella. An adversary called multiple sclerosis, a very real adversary that is the embodiment of what Kyle Reese spoke about in *The Terminator*: "It is out there, it can't be bargained with, it can't be reasoned with, it doesn't feel pity or remorse or fear, and it absolutely will not stop . . . EVER, until you are dead!"

Eretria often resorted to humor to keep her spirits up. She thought to herself: *You're going to win the lottery or someone's going to pop up and say, "Here is the money. This test is now over. You passed."* No Prince Charming was there to rescue her. She eventually located an affordable basement apartment with a kitchenette. While she no longer had to worry about curveballs like where to sleep or where her next meal was coming from, multiple sclerosis offered no reprieve. Its callous cruelty continued. MS is the real-life Cruella.

Before leaving the basement, Eretria had to plan everything in her day, such as being dropped off at the front of the store so she could grab a cart that would become her walker. She had to wait for whomever dropped her off to pick her up and load whatever she had bought into the car for her. Despite everything, Eritrea would not allow MS to take her dignity. Once a male assailant put a gun to her head and demanded money. She did not surrender or back down. She looked straight into his eyes and said, "Look at me. I can hardly walk. Go ahead, put me out of misery, pull the trigger, shoot me!"

The assailant backed up in shock and walked away. Ernest Hemingway once defined courage as "grace under pressure." This five-foot, five-inch, 107-pound girl had more courage than any UFC fighter walking into the octagon. It did not help or make her feel better when people in the store gave her "pity looks."

Eventually, it became too difficult and complicated for Eretria to go to a store. In order to cross her legs, she had to lift a leg with both hands. Her basement refuge was turning into her prison. Her biggest daily accomplishment was taking a shower and brushing her teeth. For her, that was a successful day. She is a beautiful woman and always maintained her hygiene, no matter how multiple sclerosis perverted and twisted her life. To remind herself what life should be like, she ripped out pictures of women in high heels from magazines and taped them up in the basement. She swore to herself that one day she would walk in high heels again.

She told herself: *I am not in control of the hand dealt to me by life, but I am going to play the hell out of it.* She would not give up. She was not going down without a fight. Eretria started calling and emailing everyone and every institution she could think of. She emailed the Mayo Clinic, and someone from there called her back. They told her about hematopoietic stem cell transplants (HSCT) and where to go. Eretria broke into tears and immediately called me.

She asked her neurologist about HSCT. He told her, "I wouldn't do it—there could be complications and you could die." Eretria thought to herself: *It's easy to dispense advice when you're not the one in the arena getting your ass kicked. My life sucks. I have nothing to lose.*

She remembers that we gave her a calendar of treatments and told her what to expect. It was the first time anybody had given her a plan, told her how and when things would happen, and let her know what to expect. For the first time, she felt as though a coach was in her corner.

After HSCT, Eretria stopped all medications. She got her life back. Now she can do those little things in life that the rest of us take for granted. She can go up and down stairs with a bag of groceries without hanging on to the railing and trying to hike her leg up onto the next stairway step. She can go for walks. She can go out to dinner with girlfriends. She started driving again, and she started dating again. A year after HSCT, she emailed me a video of herself running for the first time in years. She now exercises several hours a day.

When I was writing this book, Eretria commented, "Since the transplant, I am in the best shape of my life." She added, "You have to advocate for your health. Do not let someone else do it for you. And no matter how bad and hopeless it gets, never, never, never give up." On her last (five-year) clinic visit, she was in high heels and looked like a model in the *Cosmopolitan* magazine she is once again reading. Striking her at age twenty-one, MS robbed Eretria of a modeling career. On her last clinic visit, she hugged me with warm gratitude, stopping her embrace only to say, "You have no idea what a gift it is to get a second chance at life. Thank you." As of the writing of this book, she has remained free from MS and MS drugs for ten years.

Epistemology is the study of knowledge. What is true knowledge? How does it come about? What are the limits of human knowledge? In *The Glass Bead Game*, Hermann Hesse interpreted true knowledge as an intellectual, mind-driven academic gymnastic exercise. In contrast, Siddhartha interpreted true knowledge as arising from self-educated, common sense-derived experiences. I will always remember how Eretria spontaneously and succinctly summarized knowledge: "There are two types of people. There are the ones in the arena getting their ass kicked, and then there are the spectator critics in their big offices or on their big sofas. People really don't get things or understand things or agree with things until they are personally affected themselves, until life throws them into the arena." Eretria had been in the arena. She had battled the real Cruella for years. She was alone but she never, never, never gave up. In the last round of a real-life fight to the death, Eretria KOed (knocked out) Cruella.

What is HSCT? Have other patients with MS had HSCT? Did they benefit? Does HSCT work for other autoimmune diseases? How was HSCT discovered and developed for MS and other autoimmune diseases? Is HSCT safe? What is the difference between myeloablative and nonmyeloablative HSCT? Why haven't I heard about HSCT for MS or other autoimmune diseases? Why can't I get HSCT?

If you want to know, keep reading.

CHAPTER 2

WHY HEMATOPOIETIC STEM CELL TRANSPLANTATION?

When I was doing a fellowship in oncology (cancer) at the National Institutes of Health in Bethesda, Maryland, I did not particularly enjoy what I was being taught. Treating cancer with chemotherapy is, in reality, the art of infusing a poison into a patient's body to kill the cancer cells but adjusting (titrating) the drugs to avoid killing your patient. Once the cancer was metastatic, that is, beyond the site of local origin, the cure rate using chemotherapy for most solid tumors in adults was low to dismal, and toxicity from chemotherapy was high.

When compared to treating solid tumors, chemotherapy was far more effective for blood cancers such as leukemias and lymphomas, especially chemotherapy followed by hematopoietic stem cell transplantation (HSCT). For HSCT, chemotherapy is given at such high doses that the leukemia cells die, but the side effect is that the bone marrow (i.e., the blood cell-making factory inside the bones) also dies. In order to prevent permanent marrow failure (and death from lack of cells that normally circulate in the blood) you must give the patient back their own (autologous) blood (hematopoietic) stem cells or another person's (allogeneic) blood stem cells. It is for this reason that the procedure is referred to as a "transplant" or HSCT. While the future may look back in horror at the barbarism of infusing poisons into a person, this practice must be put into context. It was, in some cases, the only effective tool we had, and it does work in curing otherwise lethal leukemias and lymphomas and inducing many years of disease remissions in other cancers (e.g., multiple myeloma).

Why did I gravitate toward this treatment and then spend a career perfecting it to be safer so it could be used to treat autoimmune diseases? Events early in one's life may subconsciously affect future actions. I wonder if that was the case for myself.

I grew up in Montana and attended Hawthorne Elementary, a small country school on the outskirts of a small town. It was a wooden building with two rooms, one for first grade and one for second grade. In the basement was a kitchen where we would stand in line for lunch. Our life consisted of the classroom, the basement lunchroom, and the playground. There was no boundary to the playground, just open fields and a dirt road where yellow school buses dropped us off each morning and took us home each afternoon. The buses did not take students to their houses. They dropped you off at a "bus stop" from which you would walk home. The bus stop was just that—the place where the bus stopped. There was no bus stop shelter or identifying marker.

From the bus stop to home was about a one-mile walk down a dirt road, over an irrigation ditch, across a field, and over barbed wire fences. The irrigation ditch was too wide to jump over and too deep to cross without using a wooden plank as a bridge. The water underneath swirled like a rapid. It felt like walking the plank of a pirate's ship. I was always attentive to keep my balance as I did not know how to swim. Others had longer treks to and from their bus stop. Once

I got off the bus with a friend at his stop—it was a five-mile walk to his house.

Across the playground was a second, slightly larger wooden building with two rooms, one for third grade and one for fourth grade. It had a bell tower, and the teachers would allow a fourth grader to ring the bell to signal the end of recess. This was an experience every fourth grader looked forward to. You sounded the bell by pulling its rope down and then, as the bell swung up and you hung on to the rope, you would be pulled up into the air, temporarily free of gravity, catapulting toward the sky, before oscillating back to earth.

We would all line up in single column and wait for the teachers to give us permission to enter the classroom. As first and second graders, we impatiently awaited graduation to the bell tower building. As Rumi, the author of *Emerald Companion*, a book of prose on solitude, wrote: "Strange is our notion of freedom. For children seek adulthood. And adults, their inner child."

During third grade, one girl stopped coming to class. Her desk stood silently empty, a reminder that spoke of her absence. One day, our teacher told us that she had been sick but would be back tomorrow, and that we should welcome her. A simple explanation that seemed adequate since children tend to trust adults without need for clarification.

She returned for a total of three days. Nobody gave an explanation as to why she had been absent. When recess was over and the bell sounded, she lined up directly in front of me, and I asked her, "Where have you been?" She turned around, wearing a short black skirt that fluttered in the cool autumn breeze with a cap covering her head. Her right hand was holding a cross that was on her necklace. She looked into my eyes and then glanced away, saying, "I was sick, but I am OK now." Her smile quivered at the corner of her mouth, her hand nervously rubbed the cross over her chest, her cheeks were swollen, her eyes became lost in the distance. I asked no more questions.

After that day, she never returned. One month later our teacher started class by saying that our classmate had been suffering from leukemia and had gone on to heaven. The rest of the year her desk sat empty. I do not remember much else from third grade. The school and playground are no longer physically there, but the memory of her standing in line in front of me, so bravely scared, remains imprinted in my mind. She is still there—for me, that place and time never vanished. Today I understand that her puffy cheeks were the result of steroid treatments.

I doubt that most people, including myself, are aware of what subconsciously motivates the so-often-circuitous route of life's path, but as I reflect back to that day on the playground, I wonder if this experience fueled my passion for HSCT. Did knowing this girl in elementary school and later watching the suffering of other young patients with multiple sclerosis or scleroderma, who like this third-grade girl could not be cured, start the gears turning in my mind to apply HSCT to autoimmune diseases? Was I subconsciously trying to go back in time to help her? Perhaps that is a stretch, but I can say that the birth of this idea came with a burning passion to make it happen.

CHAPTER 3

INTRODUCTION TO HSCT FOR AUTOIMMUNE DISEASES

Turning Chronic Autoimmune Diseases into One-Time Reversible Illnesses

There has been a revolution in treating autoimmune diseases. A treatment can now convert a chronic autoimmune disease into a one-time reversible disorder. This approach was developed outside traditional trials driven by pharmaceutical companies. In developing this approach, there was never an interest, attempt, or desire to obtain a profitable patent or license. It was undertaken in an academic spirit to help patients.

It was also developed outside of the usual medical departments or medical divisions that treat autoimmune diseases. For example, multiple sclerosis, systemic sclerosis, and Crohn's disease are in the departments of neurology, rheumatology, and gastroenterology, respectively. Yet none of those departments originated, actively advocated for, or drove this advance. Medicine has become divided into subspecialties, but as the father of anatomy, Rudolf Virchow, said, "A good doctor treats the disease. A great doctor treats the patient."

My aim in writing this book is to disseminate information to the lay public, to patients with autoimmune diseases, to their family and friends, and to society. In this book, I discuss from a patient's perspective the development of hematopoietic stem cell transplantation (HSCT) for multiple sclerosis, systemic sclerosis (scleroderma), neuromyelitis optics (Devic syndrome), chronic inflammatory demyelinating polyradiculoneuropathy (CIDP), and Crohn's disease. Time and word limit would not permit inclusion of systemic lupus erythematosus (SLE, or simply, lupus), rheumatoid arthritis, diabetes, or stiff person syndrome (SPS).

The success of the HSCT treatment requires an individualized approach to each disease, which includes developing different immune conditioning regimens (which cause an immune reset) and understanding proper patient selection. When these concepts are perfected, often through trial and error and gut instinct, patients' lives can be fundamentally improved and returned to normal.

I have written and edited several medical textbooks, most recently *Hematopoietic Stem Cell Transplantation and Cellular Therapies for Autoimmune Diseases*,[1] given innumerable talks on the topic, published multiple peer reviewed articles, and set up an educational website (www.astemcelljourney.com), yet traditional medicine and most patients remain unaware that chronic autoimmune diseases can be turned into one-time reversible illnesses. *This is not a dream.* It is a hard-fought reality as these patients' stories attest.

I have omitted mention of obstacles that could be viewed as individually petty or malicious as these occur in everyone's life and should not detour or sidetrack one from focusing on constructive thoughts and positive outcomes. Alice Wine's influential 1960s lyrics direct, "Keep Your Eyes on the Prize." The prize is converting a chronic autoimmune disease into a one-time reversible illness. Rather than individuals or personalities, I will mention unintentional consequences of structural problems inherent within the medical system that have retarded its development. For example, autoimmune disease specialists do not know, perform, or understand this therapy (HSCT) and are therefore reluctant to refer patients to try it. Hematopoietic stem cell transplant (HSCT) specialists who have the technical skills for this treatment are trained in the specialty of hematology (blood) or oncology (cancer) and do not know or understand autoimmune diseases.

Medicine is the interface between the humanities and science. It is for this reason that this book is written from individual patient perspectives interspersed with ongoing refinement and development of this treatment. As a pioneer in the field, I have focused on my own experiences and work, but success has many fathers, and more and more physicians and researchers are committing to, undertaking, and contributing to this effort.

As a physician myself, patient confidentiality is a part of my existence, chiseled deep into my soul. Confidentiality is essential for patients to trust their physicians. I developed each story in this book in cooperation with each patient, who gave me written permission to include it. I omitted last names and gave all patients the option of a pseudonym for their first name. I will not provide, deny, or confirm anything about any person in this book.

In writing this book and needing to balance medical confidentiality and journalism, I have come to realize that perhaps journalism itself may benefit by adopting the medical standard of requiring written consent when releasing a person's information, or at least when quoting a person. Why not, as a journalistic profession, attempt to ensure accuracy and avoid the destructive effects of misquoting or quoting out of context?

But before starting this story, a few medical definitions may be necessary to help the nonmedical reader:

1. A **stem cell** is a cell that can reproduce itself and differentiate (mature) into other cells that can no longer replenish themselves. A stem cell is like a child who has future potential to have their own children and to grow into anything. A stem cell has not yet committed itself to a purpose or function. A mature cell has differentiated (matured), is committed to a specific function in the body, and after performing its function, it will eventually but inevitably die. It is like a highly specialized older individual who can no longer have children (unable to reproduce itself or limited ability to replicate) and who has matured to be good at a specific task in society. Most cells in our body are mature differentiated cells that have matured to make up various organs such as heart, muscle, liver, brain, gut, hair, lung, skin, teeth, bone, or to circulate in the blood as immune cells. Immune cells fight infection and determine whether an organ or tissue is self or non-self but can also attack your own tissue(s) causing an autoimmune disease.

2. There are many **types of stem cells**, some of which are present only during certain times after conception such as embryonic stem cells. In contrast adult stem cells generally exist with us throughout life in order to replenish dying or damaged mature differentiated cells. Most organs have an adult stem cell compartment for that organ. Each stem cell type has its own unique potential applications and unique problems. For this book, I refer only to the hematopoietic (blood) stem cell that is normally found in the bone marrow or blood (or umbilical cord blood) and will mature into blood cells, including immune cells.

3. The **hematopoietic stem cell** can both renew itself and become (differentiate or mature) into any type of blood cell, including red blood cells that carry oxygen to tissues, platelets

that prevent bleeding (clot blood), and immune cells that fight bacteria and viruses but also reject foreign organs and, in the case of an autoimmune disease, reject and attack one or more of an individual's own organs. Hematopoietic stem cells infused during HSCT may be autologous (collected from the patient) or may be allogeneic (collected from another person). For transplant of autoimmune diseases, almost all stem cells are autologous.

4. **Hematopoietic stem cell transplantation** (HSCT) is the intravenous infusion of hematopoietic stem cells after infusion of various drugs to destroy blood cells. HSCT has been ongoing as a standard of care since the late 1960s for leukemias (blood-derived cancers).

5. The **conditioning regimen** is the combination of agents used to eliminate the disease-causing blood or immune cells after which hematopoietic stem cells are infused. For leukemias, the disease-causing cell is often a cancerous blood stem cell. For autoimmune diseases, the disease-causing cell is often a mature immune cell derived from the blood stem cell. The conditioning regimen is a combination of agents infused usually over five to six days.

6. **Myeloablative conditioning regimen.** For cancer, the conditioning regimen is composed of agents that completely kill all hematopoietic (blood) cells, including the hematopoietic stem cells themselves. These agents are intense cancer chemotherapy drugs and/or radiation. Myeloablative conditioning regimens are designed to kill the leukemic stem cells that are causing cancer and in so doing, will kill all the hematopoietic stem cells, whether they are cancerous or normal. Hematopoietic stem cells must be infused after a myeloablative regimen or else the patient will not recover and will die from the failure to remake any blood cells. Autologous

myeloablative regimens are used for cancer. Although I do not use myeloablative conditioning regimens because I view them as too toxic, some predominately American and Canadian institutions use myeloablative cancer conditioning regimens for autoimmune diseases. Myeloablative conditioning regimens for autoimmune diseases in America are being funded by the National Institute of Allergy and Infectious Diseases (NIAID).[2]

7. **Nonmyeloablative conditioning regimen.** For autoimmune diseases, a less intense, less toxic, less expensive, and relatively more immune-specific regimen is most often utilized to eliminate the diseased immune cells. Since the hematopoietic stem cells themselves are not affected by a nonmyeloablative regimen, the patient will recover normally without infusion of hematopoietic stem cells. However, hematopoietic stem cells are infused to shorten the period required to remake circulating blood and immune cells.

8. **Common conditioning regimen drugs/agents**

    a. *Nonmyeloablative* relatively immune-specific chemotherapy examples used herein for autoimmune diseases are cyclophosphamide (Cytoxan) and/or fludarabine (Fludara).

    b. *Nonmyeloablative* biologics used herein for autoimmune disease are proteins (usually immunoglobulins that are also referred to as biologics or antibodies) that specifically target immune cells such as anti-thymocyte globulin (ATG), rituximab (Rituxan), or alemtuzumab (Lemtrada).

    c. *Myeloablative* nonimmune-specific cancer chemotherapy is used by some physicians for autoimmune diseases (but not by me) and includes busulfan or a combination of drugs called BEAM, which stands for the four myeloablative chemotherapy drugs carmustine, etoposide, cytarabine, and melphalan.

    d. *Myeloablative* irradiation is used for autoimmune diseases by some physicians (but not by me) in the form of total body irradiation (TBI)—that is, radiation X-rays that cover or bathe the entire body in radiation from head to toe. (Irradiation is the act of applying radiation.)

The take-home point is that all drugs are toxins, and myeloablative chemotherapy and total body irradiation are extremophilic poisons. It is for this reason that I advocate making HSCT for autoimmune diseases as safe and immune-specific as possible, and why I use only nonmyeloablative regimens specifically designed for each autoimmune disease.

It is important to emphasize (and reemphasize) that the autologous hematopoietic stem cell has no therapeutic effect by itself. It is infused to prevent death from marrow failure (failure of blood cells to recover) after a myeloablative conditioning regimen or to shorten the period of low blood counts after a nonmyeloablative regimen. After a nonmyeloablative regimen, hematopoietic stem cell infusion is optional but still a prudent safety precaution. The therapeutic efficacy and toxicity of autologous HSCT for autoimmune diseases is derived from the conditioning regimen (and patient selection). The autologous hematopoietic stem cells are simply a supportive blood transfusion. For a video explanation and understanding of HSCT for autoimmune diseases, please watch "This Is a Big Day" at https://astemcelljourney.com/reflect/purpose/.

I have written this book because I want patients with these diseases—not just medical professionals—to know, to be informed, and to be equipped to decide. It is your body. It is your decision. I add the important caveat that this book is intended to be educational and informational but should not replace your doctor's advice. Each patient's circumstances are unique, and yours are best known and understood by your local physician.

I am continually impressed by and grateful to all my patients, including those not mentioned in this book. All my patients sacrificed to bring this knowledge to other patients. Their experiences and lives are unique and invaluable. As Shakespeare said, "All the world's a stage." We all have a role to play. My patients were the ones on the stage.

CHAPTER 4

MULTIPLE SCLEROSIS: LOSING WHO YOU ARE

When I was a fellow at the National Institutes of Health in Bethesda, Maryland, I requested and was granted permission to learn hematopoietic stem cell transplantation (HSCT) for leukemias at both Johns Hopkins in Baltimore, Maryland, and the Fred Hutchinson Cancer Center in Seattle, Washington. For three months, early every morning I drove from Bethesda to Baltimore and then every night drove the thirty-four miles of freeway home. For another three months, I lived in a one-room studio in Seattle, just a few blocks from the Fred Hutchinson Cancer Center, where I would walk to and from each day.

Both centers had pioneered HSCT for leukemia treatment in the United States. Fred Hutchinson, under Donnall Thomas, advocated total body irradiation (TBI) as a part of the transplant regimen in order to destroy the leukemia. Well-deserved and perhaps in part for the hardship and courage required to develop a stand-alone independent center, Donnall Thomas received the Nobel Prize in Physiology or Medicine in 1990 for HSCT of leukemia.[1]

Johns Hopkins, under researcher George Santos, pioneered a chemotherapy-only approach. I loved the experience and people at both centers. But I gravitated toward the safer nonradiation approach developed at Johns Hopkins. This difference in conditioning-regimen philosophy has carried forth to this day into the field of HSCT for autoimmune diseases.

People with chronic diseases are frequently treated with drugs for the rest of their lives. Drugs, while often remarkable in the short term, when prescribed chronically seem to have lulled our medical system into an all-knowing complacency while simultaneously locking the patient into both drug and doctor dependency. Even with cancer, where the goal is to cure, chemotherapy is often scheduled to be infused intermittently over prolonged time intervals.

At that time, HSCT was an approach in sharp contrast to the status quo. It was a one-time treatment that could cure leukemia, and that one-time treatment best fit my personality. I am, as I realized later, a closet surgeon. I want to treat and fix the problem once and for all. To perform a stem cell transplant, you had to be good at everything, especially critical care. At both Johns Hopkins and Fred Hutchinson, if needed, they would intubate and administer blood vasopressors drips at the bedside, turning the treatment room into a medical intensive care unit under their control. You stayed with your patient during treatment, and that also became my philosophy.

Times have changed. Current medical intensive care unit (MICU) physicians often rotate off after two weeks, with different physicians covering during the weekends. But in the days of my transplant training, physicians in the bone marrow transplant (BMT) unit would stay at least an entire month on service. Professor William Burns at Hopkins, one of my mentors, would bring a cot to his basement office to sleep on during the night so he could be at a patient's bedside in the event of an emergency. If trouble arose, you did not transfer a patient to a general medical intensive care unit. You kept your patient. In those days, you would not consider transferring the care of your patient to another service or team not specifically trained in transplantation. And that also fit my personality.

In the 1990s, when patients returned for routine follow-up evaluations after stem cell transplants for leukemia, I noticed that they were being reimmunized with childhood vaccines such as measles, mumps, and rubella. After HSCT, the patients had lost immune responsiveness to the vaccines. It occurred to me that you want the same thing to happen in autoimmune diseases; that is, you want to lose your immune response—not to a vaccine but to your own self-proteins that your body's immune system is attacking.

My outpatient attending, Professor William Burns, was sitting directly across from me at a table in clinic, so I said in a questioning tone, "We are revaccinating these patients after HSCT?"—an obvious and, taken by itself, dumb statement made in the middle of a busy clinic. Professor Burns was too polite to act annoyed but too busy to respond. I followed up: "This means patients have lost their memory immune response." I knew my voice registered with Professor Burns, but he still did not respond. He was not ghosting me. He was just being polite, allowing me to lead the conversation to a hopefully meaningful conclusion. Then I said, "This means that we could use HSCT as treatment for autoimmune disease to make the patient lose immune reactivity to self."

Professor Burns stopped, put his pen down, and looked up, his pupils appearing above the rim of his classes that were resting low on his nose, and said, "Yes, we could use HSCT to treat multiple sclerosis." And so the idea of HSCT for multiple sclerosis (MS) began. Over time, my relationship with Professor Burns transitioned, going from professor, to adviser, to friend, and finally to an experienced and sage older brother.

Multiple sclerosis (MS) is an immune-mediated destruction of the myelin that surrounds and protects neurons within the brain and spinal cord, and which are together called the central nervous system. When the myelin is destroyed, the neurons become dysfunctional and begin to degenerate. MS begins (in 90 percent of cases) as a relatively reversible demyelinating disease that is called relapsing remitting MS (RRMS) but that in many cases over time (from a few years to several decades) will become a neurodegenerative disease called secondary progressive MS (SPMS). SPMS is degenerative and irreversible.

The central nervous system provides the essence of who we are. It allows us to walk, run, talk, balance, coordinate hand dexterity, and control the bladder; to sense our environment through hearing, sight, smell, taste, feeling, and touch; and to think, remember, and recognize our environment. As the French philosopher René Descartes said, "I think, therefore I am." When the central nervous system is destroyed, you no longer exist. Destroy any part of the central nervous system and a part of you disappears.

After my six-month transplant fellowship, I returned to the National Institutes of Health (NIH) and promptly beseeched Arthur Nienhuis, MD, Chief of the Molecular and Clinical Hematology Branch at the NIH and my boss, for a continuation of my work in Professor Burns's laboratory on HSCT for autoimmune diseases at Johns Hopkins. Nobody had previously asked Dr. Nienhuis if they could work at another center while remaining in his fellowship program (and on his payroll). The ideal embodiment of academia, Dr. Nienhuis was not offended that I wanted to use their fellowship slot to work at another institution. Instead, he expressed concern for my welfare. After I explained my idea, he cautioned that nobody at the NIH was doing work on HSCT for autoimmune diseases and told me that an academic career was best started by getting into a productive, established senior scientist's lab within the NIH.

Without hesitation and, in retrospect, audaciously, I responded that I did not want to work on someone else's project. I wanted to work on my own idea, and even if it failed with no publications, I would prefer following my instincts rather than being guaranteed publications by doing someone else's project that did not really interest me. I felt I would regret taking the safe path most often traveled in order to build a traditional academic career.

Dr. Nienhuis, a gene therapy pioneer and the editor of the medical journal *Blood*, leaned back in his chair and clasped his hands over his slightly protruding belly. He could have thrown me out of his office, but in unspoken words, I realized that above all, he respected a curious mind and scientific inquiry and knew that change often comes out of left field from young people with unconventional ideas. He tolerated, and I think secretly respected, my boldness. He paused and then told me that as long as I did one day of clinic a week at the NIH in Bethesda, I could do my research project at Johns Hopkins in Baltimore.

When I entered Dr. Nienhuis's office with this proposal, I knew it was a long-shot request, but he granted my wish. He allowed me to work at another institution, Johns Hopkins, while his branch paid my salary. This is the difference between academics versus employment by a corporation. For academics to succeed in its mission, you need freedom. Thus began my thirty-plus-year trek into the wilderness of a nonexistent field that, at the time, was sketched only in my own mind.

Back at Johns Hopkins, I was anxious to start on a clinical protocol immediately, but Professor Burns clipped my wings. From experience and wisdom, he knew the right path to take and advised me to slow down and to start with preclinical proof of principle in a mouse model of MS. I had never even heard that a mouse could get MS. I trusted Professor Burns; he knew that HSCT would not be easily accepted by traditionalists, and time proved him right. The more foundation I laid before starting human treatments, the stronger my defense would be against the harsh criticism that would follow.

I began my idea of treating MS with HSCT in the most circuitous path, reading up on and studying animal models of multiple sclerosis and other autoimmune diseases. Years of preclinical research was the Hopkins way, and that was to become my way.

But this took me down a road I wished to avoid because I support animal rights. Animals are cognitive beings. They have emotions. I really disliked working on any animal, including mice. No animal can or would give consent for you to experiment on their bodies. In academia, a lot of animal research is performed. To help cure human beings of disease, biomedical animal research is necessary to understand and better treat disease. Yet I have long worried that an unwanted and unintended consequence is a weakening, at least subconsciously, of one's respect for life in general. As the Russian novelist Alexander Solzhenitsyn said: "If we stop loving animals, aren't we bound to stop loving humans too?"

When I first started, I could not bring myself to perform a mouse operation. I asked another lab member to do the procedure on my behalf. But there was no moral difference between me doing the animal surgery versus asking someone else to do it. They always obliged me, but that did not resolve my moral quandary.

One time my then-six-year-old daughter, who loved animals, was waiting for me in my office. She walked over to the lab and saw the mice in cages and asked me why they were there. I told her that I was trying to cure their multiple sclerosis. This was a true statement, but what I did not tell her is that I had caused the multiple sclerosis with a vaccine. An MS-like disease is initiated by co-injecting a myelin protein (actually a small piece or peptide of the protein) and a vaccine antigen (for example measles, mumps, tetanus, or rubella) that co-stimulates the immune system to react against the myelin (brain-tissue) protein.

I started in a basement at Johns Hopkins with an animal model of MS, experimental autoimmune encephalitis (EAE). I learned that how the immune system responds to a protein depends on how the protein is presented. A protein presented without inflammation would often induce tolerance or unresponsiveness. When a protein is accompanied by inflammation such as tissue damage or infection (that is, co-stimulation of the immune system), tolerance could be broken, and the immune system could react against that protein even if it was a normal self-protein.

HSCT is designed as a one-time, immune-based therapy. You must treat the disease while it is immune-mediated. Looking back after thirty years, this concept and model turned out to be predictive for MS. HSCT in mice worked in the early relapsing remitting phase of EAE (analogous to relapsing remitting MS) but not in the late progressive phase of EAE (analogous to secondary progressive MS).[2]

One of my nurses was equally conflicted over animal work. She believed in me and in the novel approach of HSCT to help people, but she abhorred animal experiments. I knew that her mind was also dealing with this conundrum. One day while silently walking toward a patient's room, she suddenly stopped me out of the blue and said, "If you ever do any animals larger than a mouse, I will quit." What she was telling me is that the conflict was settled in her mind, and she would stay. I understood. I agreed with her feelings. She was right in how she felt. It was a moral dilemma that I had compromised on. She had a pure soul. Because of me, she had compromised. Did I in effect corrupt her? She was an excellent nurse, and I was glad she decided to stay.

Someday, when we have a complete understanding of cellular biology, physiology, and cellular pathways and function, I have no doubt that people will look back on animal research as barbaric and immoral. They will be right, and some animal research is grotesquely wrong and abhorrent, but it is dangerous to broadly judge history from a future moral high ground that simultaneously enjoys the benefits of that research and those sacrifices.

The Hopkins stem cell physicians became my friends, especially Bill Burns, who was always available to discuss cases. George Santos, director of the Hopkins program, also became an invaluable resource of experience for me. After Bill left Hopkins and after George's retirement, and long after I left Johns Hopkins, they would come alive whenever I phoned them to discuss a patient's case. They enjoyed our conversations. For me, it was like having an encyclopedia of lifetime knowledge available.

Despite his love of transplant, Dr. Santos, with judicious advice in retirement, hesitated but then told me not to do as he had done. When I asked him what he meant, he responded, "Do not become so immersed in work that you ignore your own family." Inevitably, passion drove me to ignore his counsel during what became a thirty-five-year marathon. I learned that, if nature is to surrender some of her secrets, a price must be paid. Professor Burns and Professor Santos have long since passed away, while Dr. Nienhuis passed more recently. I never really expressed to them the depth of my appreciation or how much respect I had for them. However, I think it was understood without me saying it.

Before writing the first protocol to perform HSCT for MS, I approached Henry McFarland, Chief of the Neuroimmunology Branch of the National Institutes of Health (NIH). He was the guru on the immunology of MS with many publications in *Nature* and *Science*, considered the two most prestigious journals for any branch of science. Although I was not a neurologist, I already had data on HSCT in an animal model of MS (called experimental autoimmune encephalitis, or EAE). I presented the results in a one-on-one conversation inside his office.

Dr. McFarland's secretary sat directly outside his office, which, for all his accomplishments, was small, filled with books and publications, and only had enough room for two people. He was perhaps the world's best researcher in the immunology of MS. Getting a one-on-one meeting with him was difficult. The key was getting through to his longtime secretary, Millie. She took a liking to my persistence and arranged a meeting.

As I explained my idea and results to Dr. McFarland, a world-renowned neurologist, I remember his response was along the lines of, "If I started doing HSCT for MS, I would be running from the neurology community for the rest of my life." Why would neurologists, as a whole, react that way? Traditionally, neurologists would treat a patient who was relapsing with steroids given to them as an outpatient. By the late 1990s, the first treatment other than steroids, which was called interferon, became available for chronic outpatient injections. This treatment, while chronic and not curative, had low risk of toxicity. On the other hand, myeloablative HSCT, as it was being performed in leukemia and other cancers at that time, was an inpatient treatment with toxicity and potential mortality. HSCT would strike a neurologist as too toxic. I, on the other hand, was experienced in doing HSCT for leukemias and cancers. I was also an unknown entity and, not being a neurologist, was less likely to be deterred by subspecialty dogma or community reaction. It is hard to expel or ostracize someone who is not a part of the community.

Dr. McFarland also warned me that many talented people had tried and failed in their quest to cure MS, but he was intrigued by my concept. He introduced me to Dr. Jerry Wolinsky from the University of Texas, who was a guru in magnetic resonance imaging (MRI), which is a technique of imaging the brain for evidence of MS lesions. One of the advantages of being at the NIH was having the opportunity to tap into the thoughts and experiences of the best minds in their fields.

Dr. McFarland's warning was true. Most of the neurology world thought I was crazy, and, at best, they ignored me. In a sense, they were right that one had to be unconventional to tackle this disease without any training in neurology. If successful, it would be a Joan of Arc–like move.

Joan of Arc was a woman with no military training who took command of the French army and altered the tide of battle in France's Hundred Years' War against Britain. To the French, she became their patron saint, but to the British, she was a despised witch. When Britain lost France, it turned toward the sea and became the largest naval empire in the history of the world. One determined woman significantly altered the history of France and Britain and accelerated the Age of Discovery. The price that nature extracted from her was a betrayal by her own jealous French king. She was burned alive at the age of nineteen in Rouen, France, on May 30, 1431. That king has long since been forgotten, while Joan of Arc remains the heroine of France to this day.

I began to release this heretical concept of HSCT for MS to the world by presenting a poster (a 48- x 60-inch printed presentation) on stem cell transplant for the animal model of MS (EAE) at the European Bone Marrow Transplant (EBMT) annual meeting in Harrogate, UK, in 1994. Because transplant was focused on leukemia, nobody paid me much notice. An exception was Professor John Goldman, editor of the journal *Bone Marrow Transplantation* and professor at the Imperial College of London, UK. Standing by my poster, this tall, thin man with a graying, receding hairline and glasses resting on his forehead remarked, "If I had MS, I would want a transplant." On the spot, he asked me to write an editorial for his journal, which was opening the door, at least in the transplant world, that I had been hoping for. Professor Goldman was a leader in the field of transplantation whom I admired. In academia, the best compliment you can give someone is respect for their work.

While doing bench research and gaining knowledge on the interaction of the central nervous system and immune system had guided me and provided a preclinical foundation, for a decade I had been unable to break out of transplanting animal models of MS (EAE and another model called TMEV). From the beginning, my goal had been to extend this therapy to patients with MS.

My resolve was strengthened when by fortuitous circumstances, I had dinner with three deities (all professors) in the field of stem cell transplantation for leukemia: Alberto Marmont from Italy, Dick van Bekkum from the Netherlands, and Shimon Slavin from Israel. I was grateful to realize that they thought similarly to me. It gave me hope that I was not alone, and that I was not crazy. From their own experiences, they all knew the obstacles that lay ahead would be hard, and they all encouraged me and shared their own experiences over dinner and wine. They became lifelong, admired friends.

Professor Marmont was a former president of the EBMT (1986–1988) who in retirement had organized the world's first stem cell transplant for systemic lupus erythematosus in Milan, Italy. He had a love for sailing off the coast of the Italian Riviera and invited me to join him. I was so focused on my work that it never came about, but now that he is gone, I regret that it will never happen.

Professor van Bekkum was an original pioneer in the field of radiation biology and was nominated for the Nobel Prize on several occasions. At dinner I learned that, despite formal retirement, he was also doing transplant in murine (mouse) models of MS and was getting results similar to mine. At another time over another dinner, he told me a captivating story from his own childhood about his family's harrowing sea evacuation from Indonesia during World War II as Japanese planes and soldiers landed and the British army was in a chaotic rout, unable to protect themselves, much less Dutch and Indonesian civilians. The ships were cramped, dark, and cold. To get as many people on as possible, personal belongings were left on the dock. Food and water were rationed. No showers were allowed, and nobody dared turn on a light at night for fear of being spotted and sunk by Japanese airplanes or submarines. Years after his passing, I was honored in 2018 with the van Bekkum Award that had been established by the European Society for Blood and Marrow Transplantation (EBMT) to honor breakthrough work in stem cell transplantation (in my case, for multiple sclerosis).

Ideas rapidly bounce back and forth in the mind of Shimon Slavin, gather momentum in a rapid stream of consciousness, and then are summarized with a clear, succinct explanation. The problem with being so far ahead of everyone is that you can shine too bright for this world to see you. Professor Slavin unselfishly gave his time to teach and educate others. Once while we sat at a table looking out over the Mediterranean he discussed his insights on immune tolerance during a meeting in Monaco, which is not exactly a cost-effective location for a society of poor researchers to meet. However, the best pastry I have ever eaten was an éclair from a small sidewalk bakery. I was taken to the bakery, whose name I can never remember, by my daughter. It is on Avenue du General de Gaulle in the French city of Beausoleil (which is adjacent to Monaco).

Most importantly, what I have learned from these mentors and other visionaries (including Professor Susumu Ikehara in Osaka, Japan, who passed away in 2021) is that people who love their work never truly retire, and despite whatever obstacle or debacle is placed in front of them, they do not complain. They continue, they overcome. It is not work. It is a passion. I also learned that nature inevitably extracts a price from you if you try to transform a thought into reality.

The First Protocol for MS

Because nobody had performed HSCT for MS, because the risks versus benefits were unclear, and because the distinction between the two MS phases—an immune-mediated early inflammatory and a later neurodegenerative pathophysiology—had not been delineated, my NIH advisors recommended that criteria for HSCT enrollment be permanent baseline neurologic worsening (instead of frequent relapses) within the year prior to enrollment. Unfortunately, the selection of patients for permanent baseline neurologic worsening (and higher disability) preordained this initial trial to selection of secondary progressive MS (SPMS) and thus to failure. In other words, the disease in our first patients was already too advanced to respond to the treatment. An immune-based therapy like HSCT will not work for a nonimmune-mediated degenerative disease.

In simplified terminology, 90 percent of MS cases begin as immune-mediated relapsing-remitting MS (RRMS) that, over a period of years or decades, eventually transitions in most patients into neurodegenerative secondary-progressive MS (SPMS). During the RRMS phase, patients may recover from an acute attack with no residual disability or with some new permanent neurologic disability, but between acute attacks, disability will remain stable. In distinction, during SPMS, neurologic disability slowly worsens between acute attacks (active SPMS or aSPMS) or without further clinical acute attacks occurring (nonactive SPMS or naSPMS). As the animal model (called EAE) had predicted, HSCT works for the early immune-mediated relapsing phase. It does not work for the later neurodegenerative progressive phase, especially secondary progressive MS, without new enhancing lesions within the prior year called nonactive secondary progressive MS (naSPMS).[3]

We Become Birds

Linda was the very first patient in America who was treated with HSCT for MS. She had two PhD doctorates: one in biology and the other in the study of birds (ornithology). She had published numerous articles, had been honored as "Woman of the Year" in 1978, and had published two books of poetry. She loved the outdoors and was a champion of the environment, animals, birds, and beauty in all of life's forms.

At the time of her transplant, having been diagnosed only five years earlier, Linda had entered the progressive stage of MS. She was unable to move her left leg, could not feed herself due to severe tremors in her hands, had slurred speech, could not get out of bed, and needed assistance to toilet herself. Her disease had left numerous areas of permanent and irreversible brain damage known as black holes on her brain scan, i.e., MRI (magnetic resonance imaging). These are appropriately named because like an astronomical black hole, there appears to be no escape once you are there.

While a tremor caused a facial quiver, Linda had a broad smile that MS could not suppress. She was not going to give up. Stem cell transplant was her last hope. Every morning during the transplant procedures, she smiled whenever anyone entered her room.

Being the first HSCT for MS in America and the second in the world (the first was performed in Thessaloniki, Greece, by my friend and colleague Professor Athanasios Fassas), the tension in the air could be cut with a knife. I remained available 24/7 and slept one block away. Fortunately, Linda tolerated the procedure uneventfully.

At first, there were some encouraging subtle improvements in her condition, but those did not last long. The transplant did not help her. It was a Hail Mary pass by us and a determined last stand in the end zone by her, but it was too late for an immune-based therapy to help what was a progressive degenerative disease. For neurodegenerative diseases, nothing helped then, nor does it to this day.

Due to the love and support of her mother, father, brother, sister, aunts, uncles, nieces, nephews, and cousins, Linda continued to receive care at home and, toward the end, in a nursing facility. Her family, especially her sister, bathed her, cut her hair, and cleaned her home. They all stayed with her and did their parts to care for her. Eight years after HSCT, Linda passed away.

Imagine the loneliness of being jailed inside a body that will not move, unable to get out of bed. It is no longer your body. It is an alien prison. Imagine the frustration of a family who loved her and remembered how healthy she had been growing up. Linda's life as she had known it had vanished like smoke in the wind. She had done no harm to anyone but was condemned to endure a torturous solitary confinement far worse than any prison sentence adjudicated to any criminal.

Her family carried her burden. The pain had left a numbing vacuum. Linda was gone. They had watched her die a little more each day. Some people have told me that MS is not severe enough to justify HSCT if it's performed earlier in its disease course. Let them say this after being sentenced to live in her body, even if only for one day.

The medical field failed her—how could this happen in the twenty-first century? I failed her, though she was grateful that someone had tried. For me, Linda was a reaffirmation of a miraculous human spirit laid bare by absence of the clutter, noise, gossip, petty wants, and the push and shove of an everyday urban life. She fought on, walking a bleak and dark path alone. She was the ultimate Olympian, but the world did not bother to see her, to recognize her courage, to offer a medal.

Linda's last request was that in lieu of flowers, donations be given to plant trees. Her brother held concerts to help remember her and their childhood. She had been his best friend. Postmortem, he gave tribute to her with a song written by Michael Peter Smith, "We Become Birds."

The next twenty or so patients I treated were in earlier stages of secondary progressive MS, but HSCT did not reverse their neurologic disability. As we followed these patients over time, progressive disability (without relapses) continued in about half of them. Did HSCT stop progression in 50 percent and slow progression in the other 50 percent? Nobody knows. My goal had always been to reverse the disease, not to watch a patient deteriorate at a slower rate of decline.

With time, I learned the right patients to select for HSCT (relapsing remitting with frequent relapses) and developed safer treatment regimens. In Linda's failed transplant, she gave of herself so that the knowledge we gained from her situation could help the lives of others. She paid a price for all of us. She taught me, and I have tried to teach others. I hope she somehow knows this.

As the relative safety of the procedure became established, I received approval to do HSCT for a relapsing-remitting MS patient with frequent relapses despite ongoing drug therapy.

The 007 Primer

James was the last patient in this first study. He was relatively young, tall, and good-looking. James was married with small children and had worked as an executive sous chef. He had been a cook since age fifteen and had worked his way up through the culinary ranks. But MS is a condition exacerbated by heat. Working by hot stoves soon forced James to forgo employment. As the insensitive cliché goes, "If you can't stand the heat, get out of the kitchen." His circumstances were not metaphorical; they were reality. Under the unrelenting pressure of having to buy an endless supply of medical drugs without an income, James and his wife of nine years soon separated. It is easily forgotten by the healthy that unrelenting disease can be destructive both for patients and families.

James was referred to me by his local physician, whose own aunt had MS. The physician called me while James was sitting in his office. Flying in from about a thousand miles away, James was in my office the following day. In the year before his transplant, he had twelve relapses, roughly one every month despite the anti-MS drugs available at that time: Copaxone, Betaseron (an interferon), and steroids. After a year of relentless attacks, James had lost much of his short-term memory and control of his legs. His knees would buckle under him.

Within a few steps, he would fall. Due to fear of injuring himself, he rarely walked anymore. Despite what MS was doing to him, he still had retained his boyish smile of sly confidence.

The transplant was uncomplicated, but this time we performed the transplant for relapsing-remitting MS (RRMS) with frequent relapses. James's life turned around 180 degrees after the transplant. All his symptoms disappeared. Within a month he was going back to the gym. He felt normal by four weeks and began working again within several months. On return visits, his 007 Bond–like swagger and quick dry humor had returned. Nurses were drawn to his charisma and uncanny wit like a magnet. I thought he was a natural to be another Johnny Carson on *The Tonight Show*. Six years after HSCT, James remarried. His children have grown up, and a healthy James now spends recreational time playing with his grandchildren.

Twenty-one years have passed since his transplant, and during that time, he has remained off all MS drugs. His neurologic disability reversed with no further clinical or imaging evidence of new disease, and several brain and spinal lesions that were present before the transplant have vanished. Like the hidden primer (the secret key) required to decipher the encryption code in the movie *Contact*, James was the primer who confirmed what I had hoped for and why I had started this journey a decade earlier: HSCT could work for patients with relapsing-remitting MS.

There is no definition of cure for MS, but James's long-term outcome suggests that perhaps, just perhaps, if we are lucky, we could start trying to direct therapy toward that goal. Perhaps like in a *007* movie, James demonstrated that the villain could be stopped by the good side.

For this first protocol, I had used total body irradiation (TBI) in the regimen. This was the only myeloablative and the only radiation-based regimen I had ever performed, and it bothered me. I was haunted by a shadow in the back of my mind that approximately 5 percent of people who undergo TBI may develop a late leukemia or myelodysplasia from the radiation.[4] I remembered the words of Dr. Eli Glatstein, Chief of the Radiation Oncology Branch at the National Cancer Institute (NCI) at the NIH. During my fellowship, he once said, when referring to total body irradiation, that "radiation was never meant to be thrown on someone like a bucket of water." He said this in jest, but it stuck with me, nonetheless.

The Fred Hutchinson Cancer Center was pushing for a TBI-based regimen for MS, and TBI was effective for some types of leukemia that infiltrate the brain (actually, the membrane or meninges around the brain). SPMS is such a destructive disease that the risk benefit from TBI could be justified, or some may say rationalized, for a patient confined to a wheelchair if afterward the patient regained independent ambulation.

But an aggressive radiation-based transplant regimen did not work for SPMS. In contrast, it did work very well for James with aggressively relapsing MS, but I knew that I could not justify (rationalize?) using total body irradiation for patients in the relapsing-remitting phase of MS (RRMS). When a patient dies under your bedside care, their death weighs heavy on your soul. Like an old black-and-white *Twilight Zone* episode, their faces flash in front of you as you look in the morning mirror. To get these points across, I titled the published report of my first HSCT trial, "Hematopoietic stem cell transplantation for progressive multiple sclerosis: failure of a total body radiation-based regimen."

At that time, neurology journals were not interested in HSCT for MS, so I published the world's first-ever trial in *Blood*, the top journal in hematology. The inclusion of the word *failure* in the title of this first publication annoyed some of the hematologists / oncologists who were pushing aggressive cancer transplant regimens that contained total body irradiation.

I had been awarded a large contract (greater than $9 million dollars) from the National Institute of Allergy and Infectious Diseases (NIAID) to develop HSCT for autoimmune diseases. I had been arguing to avoid aggressive cancer regimens when performing HSCT for MS. After my publication of "Failure," NIAID's annoyance with me intensified. NIAID, an institute of my NIH alma mater, without saying another word, stopped including me in the meetings or phone calls on development of HSCT for MS.

From this experience, I learned the golden rule: "Whoever has the gold [money] rules." But I was also relieved to be free from the frustration and fear of being forced to treat a patient with something that I thought was too dangerous and unnecessary. I had compromised on performing experiments on animals, but I would not compromise on doing what I felt was best for patients.

NIAID viewed me as insubordinate. From my perspective, I already had animal and human data that progressive MS would not respond, and I felt that total body irradiation was not justified in terms of risk benefit for relapsing remitting MS. Most importantly, I viewed myself as doing the right thing for patients. My publication of this trial with "failure" in the title did do what I wanted. It put an end to the use of total body irradiation in the conditioning regimen for MS. It forced NIAID to shift toward a less intense regimen without radiation called BEAM. This was only a partial victory, as BEAM is still an aggressive myeloablative cancer regimen.

On the other hand, when I presented these failed data at the American Academy of Neurology, many neurologists thanked me for the courage to present negative data, as a failed trial, more often than not, is never published. Who wants their name attached to failure? It is a general truism that failure is an unclaimed orphan.

In my mind, negative results can be more informative than a positive trial, and I wanted the community as a whole to know that this approach did not work in late progressive MS and, except for a very rare rapidly aggressive case of relapsing-remitting MS, as was the case for James, this regimen would be too toxic a treatment for most patients with relapsing-remitting MS.

What I knew from the mouse model and James's outcome in this first trial was that this treatment (HSCT) worked in relapsing-remitting MS. I needed to determine whether a less intense and milder noncancer (nonmyeloablative) conditioning regimen without risk or with minimal risk of late cancer could also be effective.

The Second Protocol

Scientifically, it is a fallacy to base conclusions on one patient, but James responded exactly like the mice with relapsing EAE in studies that had been done a decade earlier. Inside myself my instinct was crystal clear: this approach should be broadened to include patients with RRMS. I just needed a safer, noncancer conditioning regimen without the risk associated with an aggressive myeloablation regimen or from the multitude of total body irradiation-induced side effects such as cancer.

For this second study, I chose Cytoxan (cyclophosphamide) and alemtuzumab. As a side note, medications often have at least two or more names: a generic (chemical) name and one or more brand names and/or a trade name. The generic drug cyclophosphamide has brand names of Cytoxan and Neosar. The generic drug alemtuzumab has the trade name Campath and the brand name Lemtrada. Throughout this text, I will generally stick to one name for a drug. Due to its targeting of lymphocytes, Cytoxan had long been utilized to suppress many types of autoimmune diseases. Intravenous Cytoxan, given off-label by intravenous pulsing—albeit at doses lower than used for HSCT—had been used with benefit for RRMS.[5] Cytoxan has no patent protection, so it is dirt cheap compared to drugs that are patent protected. Alemtuzumab had just recently been approved by the FDA for treating MS. It specifically targeted lymphocytes (immune cells).

Without patent protection, no company or individual wastes time and effort for zero financial reward. No sane person would work for free, right? Yet in medicine, there are still doctors who do, working long hours to write protocols, get regulatory approval, collect and record data, report to regulatory agencies, write up results, and suffer through peer reviews to publish data with no financial, institutional, or outside financial or staffing support.

The reward lies in the less tangible asset of academic achievement. The triple threat of "patient care, research, and teaching" was the ideal of physicians when I started medical school. In this new era of monitoring productivity by relative value units (RVUs)—i.e., "money billed"—doctors are being separated and herded into either the path of clinical revenue generation as a business enterprise or a separate path of doing basic research and obtaining grant funding for the university that usually extracts 50–70 percent of any NIH award for themselves to cover their "indirect costs." Today the concept of a "triple threat" is in danger of going extinct.

For the new study using nonmyeloablative Cytoxan and alemtuzumab, I selected patients with RRMS and two or more relapses in one year before HSCT despite being on an anti-MS drug.

Taurus

The first patient treated with the world's first nonmyeloablative HSCT regimen was Barry. The regimen was Cytoxan and alemtuzumab. Barry was forty-four years old, married, and had a daughter. He coached high school ice hockey and had been a collegiate hockey player himself.

Barry had had MS for eight years. When it began to affect his vision, he searched the Internet for stem cell studies. He had diplopia in both eyes, meaning he could not see with both eyes open due to blurred vision. In order to drive, read, or work, he had to cover one eye with a patch.

Barry had been working sixty hours a week, but instead of eating lunch with his colleagues, he would go home to sleep for one hour due to MS-related exhaustion before returning to work for the rest of the afternoon. He could walk, but his legs felt constantly numb, "like they were asleep." He could not wake them up no matter how hard he slapped them. On his first evaluation for the new protocol, he did not meet criteria and was sent home. On the second visit, he met criteria.

Because this was a new protocol, I called his wife and told her what I had told Barry: it may not work! They needed to consider that as a new protocol, there may be unknown or unexpected toxicities. I always read a patient a riot act as to why they should not get HSCT. Surprisingly to me, despite this, no patient with MS has ever said *no*. Barry's wife was adamant that she wanted what he wanted, and he wanted HSCT. As Barry clarified, "I am a Taurus, and I want to get back into the game of life."

The transplant was uncomplicated. In the twenty years since his transplant, Barry has had no symptoms and has been on no medications. His legs and vision returned to normal functioning. He went back to working sixty hours a week but no longer needed noon naps and started having lunch with his coworkers. He returned to coaching hockey and playing hockey on his own. He and his wife bought a house on a lake, and every weekend they go jet skiing, swimming, and boating.

This nonmyeloablative MS study using MS-specific drugs without radiation and without cancer-specific drugs was much less toxic. Barry became the primer that a less intense nonmyeloablative regimen could work with neurologic improvement and long-term remissions but without the late risk of total body irradiation-associated cancers. He is also the primer that the beneficial effect of a non-myeloablative HSCT can persist for more than two decades after treatment.

Gentleman's Quarterly

John is a self-made man. As his financially successful father had proudly told me, John never once asked or expected his father to provide money or pay for anything. There were no slippers coming down his father's staircase. John became successful the same way his father had, by putting his boots on every morning to climb up the stairs.

Through intelligence and hard work, John worked his way up from nothing to starting his own company. He loved the outdoors and anything to do with sports. He was a fearless skier and race car driver, flirted with extreme sports, and married an Olympian. In person, he responded to everyone as a friendly, down-to-earth, trusting, next-door neighbor would respond. You would never expect that he had his own private jet. He loved life, and his optimism and friendliness were infectious. I thought that he would fit perfectly on the cover of *GQ* (*Gentleman's Quarterly*).

When MS hit him, life as he knew it stopped. When I first met John, he had an unsteady (ataxic) gait, stumbling as if he had spent a night of celebration in a bar after winning a grand prix race. But this was no celebration, there was no alcohol, and he would not wake up in the morning with a hangover but otherwise be back to normal.

John looked at me with a broad smile and said, "I am losing my mojo." He got up for the second time in twenty minutes, staggering in a zigzag path to the restroom, like a battleship sailing left and then right to avoid a submarine locking on its position. While he was not yet incontinent, John was starting to lose control of his bladder.

His business acumen had become ingrained and innate, but his memory was fading and remembering events, appointments, topics, and deadlines were becoming difficult. The company he'd built had become a part of him, but MS was stealing it away. He worried about the welfare of all the people he had hired while building his enterprise. Possibly the final deciding factor for John in seeking a transplant was the visual attacks he was experiencing, with significant worsening of his vision after each attack.

During the transplant, he had a high fever. I remember John lying supine in bed, opening his eyes and looking up at me holding his vital signs board in my hand. He was groggy, but I knew exactly what to do and told him not to worry. He slipped off to sleep. The fever resolved. For eighteen years after HSCT, only once did his local physicians think that he may have a new lesion based on an MRI that was performed as a routine test despite him being asymptomatic. He was immediately surrounded by a team of experts and started on a new experimental drug that was stopped shortly thereafter due to its toxicity. In retrospect, the "new lesion" was deemed old and not "new." John has had no new MS lesions.

Extreme sports are now a part of John's past. But twenty years after HSCT, he continues to run recreationally, has expanded his company, walks in a straight line, and helps people who long ago lost belief in the concept of a Santa Claus–like Good Samaritan coming to their rescue. John donated a state-of-the-art, high-resolution 7 Tesla MRI to a local university to better image brain lesions. This university also was the recipient of a building donated by and named after John's family.

Tesla is a measure of magnetic field strength. It is named after the Serbian-American inventor Nikola Tesla, who is also the father of the alternating electrical current used in our wall sockets. Albert Einstein called him the smartest man alive. Elon Musk named his electric car company Tesla. Almost all MRIs are either 1.5 or 3 Tesla. When you look at the images from a 7 Tesla MRI, it is like putting on glasses and suddenly being able to accurately read the smallest numbers on an eye chart.

Yeti

Whether by chance or circumstance, or because all lives are inter-connected, years later when we had moved on to another MS study, John heard about Zac, a twenty-three-year-old young man who was afflicted with aggressive MS. He had been diagnosed two and a half years earlier and had been on Tysabri (natalizumab) since his diagno-sis. Because his disease was so aggressive from onset, his neurologist started the strongest MS drug on the market (Tysabri) at the time of his initial diagnosis. Relapses continued and at the time of transplant, Zac had numbness and tingling below both knees and in both hands. It was difficult for him to remember recent events.

Zac's life had become one of fatigue, hand tremors, and furni-ture walking—that is, holding on to the closest piece of furniture in order to move himself around the room. Years of monthly infusions of Tysabri were not helping. With any type of exercise or heat, Zac's vision would "white out," as if he were staring at a blank sheet of white paper. He gave up on school activities, including lacrosse. Before MS, he had been very interested in pursuing an engineering degree, but after the diagnosis and the uncertainty that came with it, he gave up on that route. MS had made everyday tasks considerably harder for him, both physically and mentally.

Zac and his family learned about HSCT when they were directed by a friend to John (see the prior GQ section), who informed them what transplant had done for him. When accompanying her son during evaluation for transplant, Zac's mother's valiant attempt to hide her crying was betrayed by bloodshot eyes, puffy eyelids, and sniffling from tears spilling through lacrimal ducts into nasal passages.

Over the prior two and a half years, she could only watch as MS, a camouflaged carnivore, had eaten away at her son, randomly removing a piece of him only to return later to dine on another part of his body. Her son was disappearing, and she was helpless to do anything.

Zac's insurance company initially denied the transplant. Although John never told Zac or Zac's family this, he told me that if an insurance appeal was denied, he would pay for Zac's transplant. The denial was reversed upon appeal and the insurance company paid for it. The transplant was uncomplicated.

After transplant discharge, John met up with Zac. Over coffee, John recognized that they shared a love for outdoor sports. Zac was improving and mentioned that he would soon try to ride his decade-old rusty mountain bike. The next day Zac received a call from a mountain bike store. John had bought Zac a new, top-of-the-line Yeti mountain bike, one of the best and most expensive mountain bikes on the market.

Zac is now three years post-transplant. He has no symptoms of MS and has been on no medications since the transplant. He returned to college and, at the time of this writing, is two weeks away from graduation. Since HSCT, he has had straight As in all of his classes. For the last two years, he has had a girlfriend with whom he enjoys outdoor hikes and mountain biking. Zac's mother recently sent me a card thanking me for "bringing my son back."

Gyroscope

Andy was twenty-nine years old at the time of his transplant. He had earned a degree in electrical engineering and after college had been recruited by an IT firm. Computer programming came naturally to him. He received a promotion at work and got engaged. His future seemed bright and secure.

Suddenly, Andy developed symptoms of MS and within eighteen months, he had become disabled by worsening vertigo (a sensation of spinning) and memory loss. Just sitting in a chair felt like being inside a spinning carousel, but his vertigo was worse when he was walking, so he compensated by not walking much. If a person told him three things, he could only remember one of them. He felt estranged from everyone because he could not follow a conversation for more than a few minutes. He lost his job and his fiancée. He became depressed, and doctors prescribed antidepressants, which added to his sense of isolation and alienation.

Andy's transplant was fifteen years ago. Although he has not yet been able to return to computer programming, his memory has improved. He can hold a conversation and people no longer perceive him as having any cognitive problems. His vertigo, as he said, is "a thousand times better." Since transplant, Anthony has been on no MS drugs or antidepressants and has had no new lesions appear on an MRI. He met a young woman, married her, and now has three children.

Since transplant, Andy's favorite exercise is bike riding. He participates in the MS 150, a two-day, 150-mile bike ride. His second-favorite exercise is "spinning" with a group of friends. Andy explained to me that spinning is cycling on a stationary bike at different intervals and intensities. It is perhaps ironically coincidental that one of the worst MS symptoms he experienced was vertigo (a sensation of the room spinning), and now one of his favorite exercises is called *spinning*. The difference now is that his brain, which normally receives gyroscopic orientation from the inner ear, properly aligns those signals to maintain stable balance.

All the patients in this study—indeed, all MS patients—have their own unique and heartfelt life experiences. Their lives changed after onset of MS and changed again after HSCT. While chronic pharmaceutical drugs are approved for slowing the rate of disability progression, a one-time treatment with this first nonmyeloablative transplant regimen reversed neurologic disability. After transplant, patients improved. The majority never relapsed, progressed in their disease, or had new MRI activity over the years, and as I discovered in writing this book, some have had two decades of medication-free and disease-free life.

Breaking into the Neurology World

For at least the first decade after treating MS patients by HSCT, neurology journals declined my publications in their field. I felt ostracized, but I was able to publish in hematology or transplant-specific journals. The irony is that hematologists and oncologists do not see MS patients. Although grateful for publications in my own subspecialty, in general neurologists do not read those journals.

In 2009, a neurology journal, *The Lancet Neurology*, published the results of this study for the first time.[6] While more commonly read in Europe than in America, *The Lancet Neurology* is a top-tier neurology journal. Unknown to me at the time, my approach of a nonmyeloablative conditioning regimen ended up being more accepted within medical professional circles in Europe than in America. Unlike American academia, the Europeans supported the concept of a less expensive, less toxic nonmyeloablative regimen. In America, NIAID pushed a more myeloablative, toxic, and expensive approach. As a result, over time, the Europeans, myself, and the rest of the world gravitated toward working together.

In the *Lancet* publication of the Cytoxan and alemtuzumab regimen, we reported in a minority of patients the unexpected complication of another autoimmune disease, new onset low platelets called idiopathic thrombocytopenic purpura (ITP) that usually occurred within two years after transplant. ITP results in a sudden and often dramatic drop in the number of platelet cells that clot blood. These cases of low platelets (ITP) were readily and permanently reversed with a short course of immune suppression. However, if ignored, a serious and potentially life-threatening bleed may occur.

After the first case of post-transplant low platelets (ITP), we called all patients and informed them what symptoms to watch for. Although the condition was relatively easy to reverse, I nervously visualized someone much like myself returning to work and ignoring the easy bruising of skin until suddenly dropping to the floor due to an acute and lethal bleed in the brain (intracranial hemorrhage). Once again, I needed to design a new regimen that would hopefully not be complicated by late ITP.

As it turned out, the main culprit causing ITP was alemtuzumab. Alemtuzumab is a drug approved by the Food and Drug Administration (FDA) to treat MS. When used by itself to treat MS, alemtuzumab is complicated by ITP. After an ITP-related death occurred in a patient treated in the alemtuzumab drug company trial, the drug company recommended that neurologists draw blood once every month to watch for low platelets (ITP). But that was not reassuring to me, as a patient's platelet count can precipitously fall within one week. One of my patients had a normal platelet count on a yearly visit and one week later developed ITP.

The mechanism by which alemtuzumab caused late ITP when used as a single drug (monotherapy) for MS was first brought to my attention in an "At the Limits" meeting[7] in London, UK, by Dr. David Baker. Alemtuzumab, when used as solo therapy, causes a profound immune (lymphocyte) depletion followed by rapid recovery of naïve and immature B cells (B cells make antibodies), but delayed recovery of T cells that regulate new B cell function.[8] Delayed recovery of the regulatory T cells was thought to be the cause of post-transplant low platelets (ITP). I designed a new third MS protocol in an attempt to obtain the same neurologic clinical benefits without alemtuzumab and thus without the risk of ITP.

However, even I am surprised by how well patients treated with the Cytoxan and alemtuzamb regimen have done fifteen to twenty years after treatment. MS is considered an incurable disease by the neurology community. Despite the title of this book, I had never previously used the word *cure*, but is it? Did my daydream become reality in this world? Do these long-term, twenty-year results challenge the dogma that MS is incurable?

I recall Dr. McFarland's warning when I was a fellow at the NIH (more than three decades ago) that many people have tried but all have failed to cure MS. For my personality, it is better to work hard, stay focused, and remain humble rather than get ahead of the data, a caveat that I want to remind the reader. Nevertheless, in private, when I think of these patients who have gone fifteen to twenty years without MS symptoms and on no drugs, a smile crosses my lips. This smile is deflated when I think of Linda's (my first patient with progressive MS) suffering, how we knew so little, and to this day how we can do so little for the neurodegenerative phase of MS—i.e., secondary progressive multiple sclerosis (SPMS). HSCT is an immune-based therapy and only works while MS is still inflammatory—that is, still relapsing-remitting multiple sclerosis (RRMS).

The Third Protocol

I needed a nonmyeloablative regimen that would not cause, or at least have a much lower risk of causing, ITP (low number of platelets that clot blood). Believing that the main culprit was alemtuzumab, this new protocol eliminated alemtuzumab. I substituted it with another older, less expensive, and no longer patent-protected anti-immune cell antibody called anti-thymocyte globulin (ATG).

This third protocol was a combination of Cytoxan and ATG. I chose it because it is the same nonmyeloablative regimen that has been in use since the 1960s for stem cell transplantation of aplastic anemia and thus has withstood the test of time as it is still being used to treat aplastic anemia today. Aplastic anemia is a disease where peripheral blood cells—which carry oxygen (red blood cells), stop bleeding (platelets), or fight infection (neutrophils)—fall to dangerously low

levels that are not compatible with life. Most cases of aplastic anemia are autoimmune. It occurs when a particular type of the body's
immune cells (called *lymphocytes*) attack the blood cells in the bone
marrow so the body cannot make blood cells that normally circulate
in blood vessels.

Aplastic anemia is an autoimmune disease treated by transplant,
but it had not been at the conscious forefront of hematologists (blood
doctors) to apply this technology (a transplant) to other autoimmune
diseases. Similarly, for non-hematologists, the knowledge that HSCT
can cure an autoimmune disease such as aplastic anemia did not consciously register as a procedure that could be used in other subspecialties like neurology with autoimmune diseases such as MS. How
was this overlooked? I still do not understand it. I suspect it is in
part due to medicine becoming so specialized that academicians work
in increasingly isolated and separate fields. Physicians are trained to
function as their peers do in order to avoid ridicule or, worse, a law-
suit. In clinical medical care, doctors are, after all, subject to a "jury of
peers." Peer pressure to follow the herd is the standard for acceptance
and survival. Going against the herd risks career suicide.

When I was a fellow at the NIH proposing stem cell transplants
for autoimmune diseases before anyone had actually performed one
(except for aplastic anemia), I was quizzically asked, "Why are you
wasting your career on this idea of HSCT for autoimmune diseases?"
This was the pre-social media era, and the fire in my belly made it easy
for me to excuse the comments of colleagues. Their intent was not
sarcastic; it was out of curiosity or perhaps concern for me. But it was
my idea and my career to waste. At that time academia was different;
it was not expected that I should justify myself to some standardized
mean of thinking and behavior. In the current social media climate,
intimidation by an avalanche of judgmental social media posts that
place a scarlet letter around someone's neck might have pushed me
back on to the traditional path.

I did not fear someone stealing my idea because nobody thought the idea would work, or they were at least rather skeptical. But new ideas are like planted seeds that take time to sprout and fruit. A physician who was in the fellowship program with me seemed at the time to have no particular interest one way or another in my idea or train of thought. After he left the NIH and joined Johns Hopkins, he discovered some patients with aplastic anemia without a suitable donor who had been given transplant doses of cyclophosphamide without stem cells. He tracked them down and found that their aplastic anemia had remained in a long-term remission.

This revelation prompted Johns Hopkins to start using transplant doses of Cytoxan (200 mg/kg) without anti-thymocyte globulin (ATG) and without stem cells to treat MS. Despite good initial response, the high early relapse rate meant an early end to their trial. The results of their trial told me that transplant doses of cyclophosphamide by itself were not strong enough (not immune ablative enough) for long-term remissions of multiple sclerosis. Fortunately, the regimen I settled on, Cytoxan and ATG, was effective. For optimal efficacy and minimal toxicity, the regimen needs to be tailored for each disease. Cytoxan/ATG was strong enough for RRMS.

Go, Girl, Go

Roxane was fourteen years old when she was diagnosed with multiple sclerosis (MS) in the spring of 2007. Prior to being afflicted with MS, she studied and played the piano, was a straight-A student, an avid swimmer, and a basketball and tennis player. Between studies, athletics, music, and her social life, she made time to participate in the United Nations Children's Fund (UNICEF) and overseas student conferences.

On a trip back to Iran after a student's academic competition that had taken place in India, Roxane developed excruciating daily headaches. She began to have balance problems, which affected her walking. Her graceful penmanship deteriorated to a second grader's handwriting. Eating and drinking or just holding a tennis racket or trying to dribble a basketball became next to impossible.

At the beginning, physicians attributed her symptoms to stress from being a very competitive student, until an imaging study (MRI) of her brain demonstrated demyelination in the brain's coordination center (the cerebellum). Her parents stopped their lives and flew her to the United States. Physicians at Stanford, the University of California at San Francisco (UCSF), and the University of California at Los Angeles (UCLA) hospitals all came to the same conclusion: it is multiple sclerosis.

The doctors told Roxane that she should not exert herself and that she should give up sports because her lack of balance was a danger to herself and others. One doctor told her parents that the damage to the center of her brain, along with her poor balance, may cause her to become bedridden within a couple of years. Her world was turned upside down before she could even graduate from high school. The simple but hauntingly accurate words of professional boxer Mike Tyson rang true: "Everybody has a plan until they are hit in the face."

Like a jackhammer chiseling away at her life, the physical limitations and emotional costs of MS continued to accumulate and chip away at Roxane's spirit. Through sheer determination and willpower, she graduated from her high school as valedictorian in 2010. She stumbled across the stage to give her talk to a standing ovation from the audience.

Her balance was off. She was numb in her legs and chest and could not feel her hands. Her tremor became so bad that she could not use a fork for fear of stabbing herself in the eye. Her shaking hands caused a glass of water to splatter everywhere. She could no longer hold a cup to drink. She could not run and had to hold on to another person, usually her dad, to walk. Her penmanship deteriorated to an illegible cacography of chicken scratch.

Frequent attacks of MS, the side effects of medications, and a dismal prognosis from the best California medical centers resulted in an emotional roller coaster. Roxane was extremely realistic and intelligent and knew that she was looking at a shattered and wasted life. Even though she did not know where to find help, she refused to accept that her life would be condemned to ruin by MS. Her parents knew the score, but they tried their best, were always there, and would not give up on their daughter. They searched the Internet, found patient support groups, and learned about HSCT.

They turned to California Children's Services (CCS), a state program whose mandate is to ensure that: "Children up to 21 years old can get the health care and services they need."[9]

But the state of California and CCS did the opposite. CCS actively fought to prevent Roxane from getting HSCT. The family hired a lawyer and took CCS to court, but the convoluted laws required that the matter be pursued within a CCS court. I testified on Roxane's behalf.

The system is designed so the parents had to respectfully beg a CCS judge to overturn a CCS decision being argued by a CCS lawyer; they were all on the same payroll. For everyone except those connected to CCS, which was immersed in its own game, the outcome was obvious. It was preordained. What else could one expect from a court with a self-approved internal self-conflict? Except for being state-ordained, this struck me as the definition of a kangaroo court.

To no one's surprise, the CCS court upheld CCS's refusal to provide a transplant. Afterward Roxane's mother said in frustration, "We are paying for a system to work against us." It was not the first nor the last time I have witnessed a bureaucratic system hide behind its stated credentials to add insult and injury to already-suffering patients. I remember the words of Ron Paul, a physician and US Congressman, who said, "They give laws names that are the opposite of what they really are."

When detached bureaucracy and ruling aristocracy fail a patient, it is the family and friends who ultimately find the finances through their own ingenuity and self-sacrifice. After HSCT, Roxane's neurologic improvements began immediately. She could drink from a glass. Her voice quivered less. She could walk without assistance. Out of curiosity both her UCSF and UCLA doctors wanted to see her three months after transplant. Both centers had recommended against HSCT and had thus provided ammunition for CCS without having to testify directly against their patient or be confronted with evidence to the contrary during the court hearing.

After HSCT, three UCSF physicians saw Roxane, and when her mother and Roxane beamed with optimism about the neurologic improvements, one UCSF doctor turned to the mother and said, as her mother repeated to me, "You do not know anything. MS could come back tomorrow." Roxane's mother was crushed. Her daughter had been a UCSF patient since Roxane was fourteen. Throughout that time, they had agreed to whatever UCSF requested, including their unreimbursed requests for research on her daughter's blood for genetic and immunologic studies. The family and Roxane walked out of the appointment and never again returned to UCSF.

The UCLA neurologist also evaluated Roxane after HSCT. However, after the examination, the neurologist turned to Roxane and, as her mother recalls, said, "I was wrong. I am glad you did this."

It has been more than a decade since Roxanne's transplant. Since then, she has had no relapses, no complications, and no treatments. She plays sports again and is an avid swimmer. She is normal except for diminished fine motor skills and the persistence of numbness in her right hip after walking or jogging a mile. She obtained a scholarship to attend the University of California, Berkeley; graduated with honors in American studies with a focus on American politics, technology, and society; and became a member of Phi Theta Kappa, the international college honor society. Roxane took and passed the Law

School Admission Test (LSAT) with flying colors. She was awarded a scholarship to a California law school.

After the transplant, I arranged for Roxane to speak of her journey at the Vatican in a conference in which I was a lecturer. Four years after Roxane's transplant, I published in the *Journal of the American Medical Association* (JAMA) the results of HSCT for MS on Roxane and 150 other patients.[10] My article was accompanied by a skeptical editorial from a neurologist at UCSF, where Roxane had been a patient and whose center had not supported her in the CCS appeal to provide HSCT.[11]

Suffering from MS, being told it is incurable, having the system fight against you, and then undergoing HSCT engendered Roxane with a new passion and a new compass in her life. Roxane recently told me that she is studying law because she is planning to become a health-care lawyer. I did not say anything, but I thought to myself, *Go, girl, go!*

A Place Where Sky Meets Land

When Jenny contacted me, she was a practicing physician in the United Kingdom who specialized in psychiatry. She went into psychiatry because she loved the study of the mind and human behavior.

What convinced her that she needed something more than MS drugs was a deterioration in her baseline between attacks. Between attacks, she could no longer run and was struggling to walk. She found out about HSCT from her father, who found an article about HSCT for MS in a lay magazine.

Sitting in the hospital room during transplant provided her time for contemplation. As Jenny later told me, "Most people with careers are on a treadmill and cannot get off. They become a prisoner to their success. They become their career. Illness gives you time to rethink life."

When Jenny told other physicians about HSCT for MS, the reaction she got was that it was a procedure performed in a dilapidated, dark back alley of some border town. This perception, as well as many others, contributed to her realization that many problems arise from embedded thought processes that maintain our interpretation of reality independent of the "real reality."

Jenny realized that our minds are creatures of habit. Early life conditioning creates neural pathways, which become entrenched with repetitive thoughts, leading to repetitive behaviors that cause the same patterns to play out in adult life. Ironically, having MS became her greatest teacher about neuroplasticity, the power of the mind, and self-awareness.

She discovered that she wanted to open people's minds by helping them to understand what in their minds was driving their perceptions and creating their experience of reality. She wanted to wake them up to the way or process involved in thinking itself. Jenny realized that neurologic pathways and connections may become more fluid and that, with the right questions, tools, and guidance, new connections, new perceptions, and different responses could be established.

It takes energy but the mind is plastic and can be remodeled. Thought processes can be redirected away from negative patterns and toward more joy-filled, creative experiences. It often, however, takes a traumatic life event for this to happen.

After HSCT, Jenny's neurologic function returned to normal. She is now ten years post-transplant and, in her own words, remains "perfectly normal" with no disability and no medications since transplant. She is a trail runner and regularly does yoga.

Her husband, who is from a legal and corporate background, partnered with Jenny to combine their knowledge and experience of science, psychology, and mythology to create a movement dedicated to helping people wake up to their programming and reconnect with their true nature and love of life.

Post-HSCT, Jenny and her husband discovered their love of dance and music and collected a group of scientists, musicians, behavioral experts, engineers, artists, and entrepreneurs and created a live experience called Skyland, a fusion of science and celebration in the expansive beauty of South Africa.

Jenny believes that the struggle with disease contains the seeds of transformation. Ten years post-HSCT, she says MS and the HSCT treatment and what it catalyzed in her have been the greatest gifts and teachers of her life. As American President John Adams once said, "Every problem is an opportunity in disguise."

Jenny left South Africa with her parents when she was only eight years old. She has returned to South Africa with her husband and their young daughter, who was born after transplant. Whether knowingly or perhaps instinctively, she has completed a generational life cycle.

Second Chance

"Do you have a history of neurological conditions?" Shree's neurologist asked while looking at her brain scan (MRI). Shree's mother, who spoke little English, rolled her eyes and with a smile said, "Yeah, maybe someone from the other side of the family is mental."

Jokes are a method to relieve stress, like the joke, "Cheer up, the worst is yet to come." Shree's diagnosis was multiple sclerosis, and the worst was yet to come. For over a decade, she was prescribed four different MS drugs, including Rebif, Tecfidera, Gilenya, and Tysabri. None was effective in ameliorating her symptoms. While placing Shree on these drugs, her doctors' criteria of success were simply whether new brain lesions appeared on her next brain scan—a criterion that was meaningless to Shree. She wanted her chronic severe fatigue and chronic lack of balance (ataxia) to go away. She had become dependent on a cane and wanted to walk without it again.

For Shree, living with multiple sclerosis was like living under a sword of Damocles that was hanging by a single thread, ready to drop at any moment and take away yet another part of her neurological function. Her disease relentlessly progressed with devastating impact on her emotional, professional, and financial health. Her career, which she had prioritized to the exclusion of everything else, was spiraling downward. She became dependent on a cane and was worried that she would end up in a wheelchair.

Thirteen years after her MS diagnosis, Shree took matters into her own hands and got a hematopoietic stem cell transplant (HSCT). For six years before transplant, she had been using a cane to walk. Six months after HSCT, she was walking without assistance and training for a half-marathon. One year after HSCT, she began working full time. Five drug-free years since transplant, today Shree works long hours and has the energy of her younger self.

For her, the MS decade of debilitation was also a period of deep self-reflection and personal growth. She realized there were multiple inefficiencies in the delivery of healthcare. Most importantly, she discovered she had not been made aware of any alternative treatments to the expensive drugs she was being prescribed. Also, her doctor's success criteria were not meaningful to her. Whether new brain lesions occurred was irrelevant to her quality of life. Her doctors had never discussed eliminating her symptoms. They had never discussed a return to normalcy.

Crisis brought clarity, Shree says. Through her lived experience, she has found a cause worthy of pursuit—advocacy for patients living with similar chronic conditions. "There are so many of us in the US alone," she said, referring to individuals who have no hope of cures and are dependent on expensive chronic medicines. And there are many barriers to access HSCT (further discussed in chapter 8).

Decades of professional experience in the pharmaceutical industry has afforded Shree access to world-class scientific expertise, regulatory agencies, policymakers, and industry innovators in biotechnology. Now she is leveraging these resources to grow awareness so individuals can access innovative treatments such as HCST in the community of patients with chronic or rare diseases. Shree says, "An innovative treatment gave me back my life. This second chance at life is a blessing that I want to share with others."

What Our HSCT Randomized Trial Did Differently

Despite these patient histories (and many more), despite my publications in peer-reviewed journals, and despite what my patients knew and said, I needed a randomized trial if anyone in the medical world was going to seriously acknowledge these results. I also knew and appreciated the value of a randomized trial. About two decades had passed since my original concept, and I knew that making HSCT the standard of care for RRMS would require a randomized trial.

I read every randomized trial for drugs to treat MS. Drug companies initially compared their drug (called disease-modifying therapy, or DMT) to a placebo (a sugar pill) control. Later trials compared their new drugs to the weakest drug on the market (an interferon or copaxone). Drug trials also enrolled newly diagnosed patients who had generally received no prior treatments.

A drug company spends stifling amounts of money to comply with regulations and time-consuming paperwork in the hope that its drug will get FDA approval, which will afford it an exclusive license to recover its research and development costs and make a profit for the investors and stockholders who are members of society willing to buy stock or risk investment in a start-up venture. Naturally, a company wants its trial to succeed. Why treat people already failing several DMTs who may have a disease that is harder to control? Why show that your drug is better than the best current drug or enroll treatment-refractory disease when all you need to get a license is to show that you are better than the weakest drug in treating a virgin (untreated) patient?

For MS, while there are other scales, the standard neurologic disability scale is measured (quantitated) by the EDSS (Expanded Disability Status Scale) on a scale from 0 to 10. The higher the number, the worse the neurologic disability. Zero represents a person with no neurologic disability. No pharmaceutical drug improved the EDSS (neurologic disability) in its study cohort, or if it did, it was by no more than 0.2 points.[12] This difference has no clinical meaning to an individual patient. Depending where you start on the EDSS scale, one must improve by 1.5, 1.0, or 0.5 to have a clinically meaningful and examiner-reproducible improvement.[13]

Coming from outside the field of neurology, what I learned from reading these publications is that drug company trials did not use improvement in neurologic disability as the primary endpoint because MS drugs do not improve neurologic disability in a clinically meaningful manner. Why should they make improvement in neurologic disability the primary endpoint? If they did, drug trials would be declared failures. There would be no FDA-approved drugs and no financial rewards.

Another important outcome in treating any disease (especially multiple sclerosis) with high morbidity but low mortality is improvement in quality of life. There are many scales that measure quality of life. The most common and validated measurement scale used independent of disease or illness is the short form 36 (SF-36). The SF-36 goes from 0 to 100. The best quality of life is a score of 100. Most MS drug trials did not report changes to quality of life, and those that did report had changes well below the clinically meaningful threshold change of 5 points. For a patient to feel a meaningful improvement in their quality of life, the SF-36 must improve (increase) by a minimum of 5.[14]

Because MS drugs do not cause clinically meaningful improvement in quality of life, drug company trials do not use improvement in quality of life as an endpoint. MS studies are often published in top-tier medical journals without even mentioning quality of life. Why should they do this? If they did, the study would appear to be a failure.

If drug company trials are not approved based on clinically significant improvement in neurologic disability nor on improvement in quality of life, how do they get FDA approval? In the field of MS, the primary goal for drug approval has generally been the number of acute attacks or number of new MRI lesions or worsening of neurologic progression compared to a control arm (either a placebo—a sugar pill—or, in more recent trials, a first-generation drug). The approval process is based on slowing MS disease activity and/or slowing the rate of a patient getting worse. It is not based on reversing neurologic disability or improving quality of life.

For my HSCT trials, I needed to do better. Treatment, in order to be clinically meaningful, should document significant improvement in both neurologic disability and in quality of life as endpoints. Drug trials were done on previously untreated patients. Given the inherent up-front risk of HSCT, patients with aggressive RRMS failing (relapsing) one or usually several different classes of MS drugs were selected for HSCT. While drug company trials compared their drugs either to a placebo or to the weakest MS drug, HSCT was compared to the best available drug.

Whenever designing a randomized trial, one must consider the ethical concept of equipoise (equal effect). You need a randomized trial to finally prove that the new treatment is superior. On the other hand, a physician cannot ethically give effective treatment just to one group but not the other. From our earlier experience, as noted, it certainly appeared that HSCT would be more effective. A randomized trial would not maintain equipoise unless all patients could be guaranteed the opportunity of HSCT. To achieve this, the study had to allow crossover to HSCT for those who continued to fail on the control arm.

When the effect between the two arms in a randomized trial is similar, a larger number of patients are needed to show a statistically significant difference in effect. That is why drug company trials have about 150 to 200 patients in each arm. Working from our prior non-randomized results and with a statistician, it was estimated that an HSCT randomized trial needed far fewer patients (110 patients, fifty-five in each arm) to show a significant difference which turned out to be right. I called the trial MIST (Multiple sclerosis Immune suppression versus Stem cell Transplant).[15] It compared the best available DMT (MS drug) to nonmyeloablative HSCT using a Cytoxan and ATG (anti-thymocyte globulin) conditioning regimen.

Twice

Billy was a longtime fisherman and the youngest harbormaster in the state of Massachusetts. He was responsible for the security and safe operation of the harbor at Martha's Vineyard. As time went on, things changed. His energy and drive were enigmatically disappearing. Despite not being old in physiologic years, Billy battled fatigue and exhaustion, especially during hot summer days.

Multiple times a day during the summer, he would close himself inside a walk-in freezer at the fish market. He dreaded going back out into the heat. Eventually he had to quit his dream job because every day he was too tired to meet its demands. He had mechanical, construction, and boat maintenance aptitudes and tried, from an air-conditioned office, being a contractor, building houses for a living.

That career was also derailed when he became paralyzed on one side. After a brain imaging (MRI) scan, Billy finally received a diagnosis. He suffered from multiple sclerosis.

He lived in the backyard of the medical megacomplex of Boston (Tufts Medical Center, Beth Israel Deaconess Medical Center, Brigham and Women's, Massachusetts General Hospital, and so forth) and spent years on prescription drugs while the side effects of these prescription drugs were treated by adding more drugs to his treatment plan. Billy continued having acute attacks (relapses) about every six months. He had to stop working entirely. He barely had the energy to sit up and eat the dinner that his wife cooked for them. He spent his days in a daybed in his living room with just enough energy to keep from collapsing under his own weight. He did not look like a fat, blubbery cetacean, yet every day he lay there like a beached whale.

One day a fishing colleague told him about HSCT. He sought the advice of his Cambridge, Massachusetts, neurologist, who said, "Your MS is out of control. I will not stop you." By chance, Billy went to the control arm of the randomized MIST trial—that is, more DMT drugs. He kept relapsing and, after one year of more drugs, his neurologic disability was worse. Due to continued drug failure, he crossed over and received HSCT. His transplant was uncomplicated.

After HSCT, upon returning to Boston, he restarted physical therapy. At the end of his second visit, the physical therapist said to him, "This is a game changer. Who is your doctor?" After two weeks, he started going to the YMCA for exercise. The head of the gym asked him what was happening and was so fascinated by his story that he started training him personally. Billy, who had previously been unable to stand for more than a few minutes at a time, started working out five to six days a week for a year with trainers who volunteered their assistance. He got stronger and stronger and very slowly regained his balance and coordination.

Since HSCT six years ago, he has remained free of MS drugs. Billy can walk and even run and ride a bike. With his wife, he has walked the cliffs of Cornwall and hiked in Scotland and Italy. He moved to Florida, has no heat intolerance, got a job, and is renovating an off-grid cabin for recreational use. At work, he moves refrigerators and straps bags of concrete to pallets. Despite working in the Florida heat and humidity, he has never again shut himself inside a freezer. Billy now does one hundred push-ups every morning before work.

With his newfound energy, Billy bought two boats—an 18-foot Boston Whaler and a 26-foot Panga—to explore the backwaters of the Florida Keys. He named his Boston Whaler *Twice* in honor of the second life that HSCT gave him. He wrote to me that, after the transplant, his motto became, "You only live life twice."

The Bannister Heroine

At age twenty-seven, Amanda was diagnosed with multiple sclerosis. She had been experiencing symptoms for three years before her diagnosis and was relieved to finally have an explanation for her intermittent and unpredictable numbness, fatigue, and failure of coordination. Her neurologist told her that most people with MS do well after starting MS drugs. There seemed to be no need to worry, so she started an MS medication and attempted to get on with her life.

There are no current laboratory tests or biological markers to determine if the course of MS for a patient will be mild or aggressive. The best current indicator for aggressive multiple sclerosis is to observe how it has been recently acting. MS that is having frequent relapses will generally continue to behave aggressively.

Amanda kept having flares and, despite being on MS drugs, needed steroids and intravenous immunoglobulins. Her symptoms became constant, with numbness and dysfunction of both hands and her right leg. After only four hours of work, she would go home to sleep until it was time to pick her child up from day care. Riding a bike, running, yoga—all things she enjoyed that used to be a part of her life—became too difficult to do. Piece by piece, she was losing what made herself *her*. She kept canceling engagements and plans with friends. As Ann Romney (wife of the senator and former presidential candidate Mitt Romney) once said, "MS robs you of who you are."

By summer, Amanda started to have urination and balance problems, and walking had become noticeably more troublesome. She worried about her family. What was going to happen to them? Who would take care of her child? Amanda was devastated when she learned she had been randomized to the control group. She had been randomized to standard of care—that is, to continuing more MS drugs.

Amanda traveled from *Alaska* for each evaluation and each MRI showed new lesions, but her disability had not increased when assessed by a blinded neurologist (a neurologist who does not know what treatment the patient received). She was switched to natalizumab (Tysabri), the most aggressive MS drug available at the time. She continued to relapse without abatement in frequency. It was insane to watch her relapse, but if we did not stick to the rules of the randomized study, this therapy would never be accepted. Plus, she was receiving the best standard of care drug available by the medical community at that time. In terms of ethical care, the saving grace was that I had built in a crossover arm for failure (defined by a sustained increase in neurologic disability, not by continued acute attacks).

After more than two more years of flares, steroids, new lesions, and continued MS drugs, her neurologic disability (EDSS) was sustained high enough to cross over to HSCT.

Amanda is now ten years post-transplant and no longer worries about her child's future. She had at best hoped that HSCT would stop her MS. Amanda wrote to me, "Saying that HSCT surpassed my expectations would be an understatement." Improvements began before she had even been discharged from the hospital. She never took anti-MS drugs again, nor did she need any more medication for bladder and urine problems. She no longer needs to sit to shower, can put her pants on while standing, and has returned to work full-time.

About a year and a half after HSCT, Amanda started running again, and two years after HSCT, ran the Shamrock Shuffle, a 5K race. It had snowed two feet the night before the event (it is held in Alaska), making the trail both a run and a slugfest. Upon crossing the finish line, tears welled up in her eyes and froze as they slipped down her cheeks. Before MS, she would have thought it ridiculous to cry after a three-mile race, but MS had taken away her ability to run, and she had thought it would never return. She thought she would be in a wheelchair. After HSCT, Amanda kept running and running and the next summer completed several races, including two half-marathons.

The following summer, she completed her first-ever triathlon. Every time she crossed the finish line in these competitions, tears returned to her eyes. In October 2019, she ran a marathon, a 26.2-mile race, in the city where HSCT gave her life back to her.

Amanda is now a mother who no longer worries about who will be there for her child. She told me that HSCT not only gave her life back to her, but it also gave her child back their mother.

As Amanda runs, she thinks about being told that she would never run again and about lying in a hospital bed barely able to walk. Multiple sclerosis is a chronic war. Like any war veteran who has experienced intense conflict and prolonged battles, most MS patients suffer from post-traumatic stress disorder (PTSD). HSCT is the cavalry that rescued Amanda and unlocked the secret to recovery. Although her life has returned to normal, fear that the demon called multiple sclerosis will return still haunts her. With each new race or triathlon, she buries MS deeper into its grave. That is why tears roll down her cheeks at the completion of every competition.

Roger Bannister became a hero, and rightly so, as the first man to run a mile under four minutes, once thought to be an impossible feat. Every time Amanda runs a race, she accomplishes a feat that was something hitherto also thought impossible in this world. The world does not know her accomplishment. Only Amanda, her family, and I know that she is a heroine perhaps greater than Roger Bannister— and now so do you.

Brahman

A sergeant at Fort Hood, Lee's nickname was Brahman (for Brahman bull) by his military platoon because of his physical prowess. Whenever there was something heavy to lift that normally would take two men, he would move it almost single-handedly.

Lee was diagnosed with MS shortly after returning from deployment to Kuwait. Despite taking MS drugs, within one year he had developed over seventy new lesions in his brain and had started using a cane and a walker. He was randomized to HSCT.

The transplant was uncomplicated. Neurologic recovery started before leaving the hospital. Within weeks, he was walking unassisted. He was a soldier's soldier. The Army—more accurately, his platoon— was his life. At the time when he entered the military, it scrubbed you down until you were no longer a separate individual, and then through emphasizing accountability, responsibility, hard work, perseverance, and unity, it built you back up into a cohesive unit.

Lee's physical prowess and strength returned, but since HSCT had given him a new opportunity at life, he had some decisions to make about his future. After discussing things with his wife and taking into account changes occurring within the military, he made the tough decision not to reenlist. It was time for change. He felt it. He had a new life to live.

Following HSCT, for five years Lee worked fourteen hours a day, six days a week, outdoors doing heavy work on drilling rigs. He became a roughneck who was loved by the other derrickmen on the rig. He looked out after his crew as a sergeant would for his platoon. Two years after transplant, he once again became a father. Everything was going well. He had been free of MS symptoms and drugs for five years.

At five years after HSCT, numbness occurred in his neck and several weeks later, he had to crawl up the stairs of his front porch to enter his house. He had relapsed. I was hesitant to perform a second HSCT, but Sergeant Lee was strong-willed and persuasive. And I could not let him sit in a wheelchair with his brain on fire from MS. After his second transplant, he returned to working fourteen to fifteen hours a day for six days a week on drilling rigs.

As I write this book, Lee remains in remission. When last I spoke with him, he had just returned from hunting elk in the Big-horn Mountains, hiking five miles a day while wearing a sixty-pound backpack. Despite receiving no further therapy, about 75 percent of patients do not relapse after transplant (about 23 percent relapse using this regimen—in Sergeant Lee's case, relapse occurred five years after HSCT). I have only performed a second transplant on two patients with MS who relapsed after HSCT; he was one. In both patients, the second transplant appears to have responded with a longer and ongoing second remission (when the second remission is longer than the first, it is called a remission inversion). Lee has regained his athletic, muscular prowess; imposing, tall, broad-shouldered stature; wide smile; effortless gait; and gentle nature.

A Mess

MS upended Kate's professional life as an attorney, as well as her personal and family life. Two neurologists advised her to postpone having children, as most MS drugs may injure the fetus and would need to be discontinued before pregnancy. Because MS drugs are not a cure, and because MS would be with her forever, she opted for childbirth sooner when she had less disability rather than later when disability may have further complicated pregnancy and delivery. Her MS flared while Kate was pregnant with her second child.

Mobility became a limitation to caring for her child. She was too scared to carry her daughter downstairs for fear of dropping her. Kate seldom took her daughter outside without another adult present, given that her toddler walked faster than her. If her toddler ran out into traffic, she would be unable to catch her. Eventually, Kate became unable to cross a street. Her mind would say go forward, but her body would freeze. More than once, she had to call her husband to come get her.

She began to work from home full time. She stopped traveling to her firm's office. Her firm was supportive, but she lost the opportunities for public speaking engagements, client pitches, and off-the-cuff, in-person conversations with clients, colleagues, and other lawyers. A hand tremor made it difficult for her to drink coffee without burning herself or staining her clothes. Her legs would wear out while walking through an airport. Poor bladder control alone prevented public outings. MS was isolating her, cocooning her inside her residence.

During the few years before HSCT, she was on Tecfidera, had tried Tysabri and intravenous immunoglobulins, and had had over a dozen neurologist appointments, six MRIs, and three three-day intravenous steroid treatments (to treat relapses). The MS drug Tysabri was administered intravenously at an infusion center. Arranging transportation to her treatments became incredibly time-consuming.

Kate's treatments and drugs were failing. Everything her medical team tried was failing. Psychologically, the biggest impact was that her future had become uncertain. How could her family continue to deal with this? How long before she was completely incontinent? How could she keep her family from suffering from her hardships? How long before she was in a wheelchair or became bedridden?

Throughout it all, her daughter used the mondegreen language slip of "a mess" instead of the word "MS" when talking about her mom's condition. The term *mondegreen* was coined by the American writer Sylvia Wright. It occurs when a listener does not understand or mishears something and then subconsciously substitutes a new phrase or meaning that makes sense to the situation. *A mess* was an accurate description of Kate's state.

For the first four weeks following HSCT, there was no improvement. Exhaustion, fatigue, brain fog, and gait problems in addition to nausea continued. Then nearly all at once, those symptoms just melted away. Kate could suddenly walk better. She could walk on uneven floors, walk without assistance, walk without another adult, walk around a store by herself, walk across a parking lot. She gave away her rollator walking aid. Kate still carries a collapsible cane in her purse. It is her safety net. In the six years since HSCT, she has used it once. She returned to working in her law office as well as traveling for work and pleasure and flying internationally.

Her family recently bought a new house that does not have a main floor bedroom. No main floor bedroom was a deal-breaker when they bought their previous house because Kate could not walk upstairs. Before HSCT, MS made it impossible for Kate to play the piano. She still cannot play *Capriccio Brillant*, an 1832 composition by the German pianist Felix Mendelssohn, which was the last piece she played before MS destroyed her fine hand dexterity (coordination). Kate is now playing an arrangement of Disney songs. The one she is currently relearning is "When I See an Elephant Fly." Kate is herself relearning to fly.

She still cannot run, but HSCT allowed her to regain independence, get off medications, and stop fearing her future. She wrote me that her only regret was not learning about and getting a transplant sooner.

Ali Strong

Ali worked in corporate quality assurance and was a single mom with a daughter in high school. As time progressed, she became sensitized to medications. Copaxone caused anaphylaxis, while Rebif and Avonex precipitated severe flulike symptoms that would leave her bedridden. Her neurologist was concerned about starting several newer MS medications because of her very high JC virus load.

JC virus causes a particularly virulent and too often lethal brain infection in patients with MS who stay on the MS drug natalizumab (Tysabri). The JC virus infection causes a disease called progressive multifocal leukoencephalopathy. It has also (rarely) been reported in patients receiving fingolimod (Gilenya) and rituximab (Rituxan). I would always check the JC index (the level of the virus in the blood) before a transplant just in case reactivation of the virus occurred after HSCT. It was always a dark shadow in the back of my mind as a possible complication, but it has never occurred even in patients with a very high pre-transplant JC virus level, and to date, it has not been reported to occur in the European registry with over 2,000 transplants for MS.

Patients are warned of this dangerous possible complication, and to decrease the risk of JC virus infection, we delay HSCT for variable time intervals after stopping MS drugs to clear their biologic immune suppression effects. I universally found that patients were willing to accept the possible risk of JC virus infection over continuing with the real and present danger of MS and of JC virus infection as a complication from some standard MS drugs.

MS forced Ali to stop working. Her cognition had declined. The words in her head would not come out of her mouth. She described it as if "someone had tied my tongue." During a work conversation or meeting, she could not process words and could not remember what she or others had said only a few moments earlier. People would correct her for repeating the same phrase that she had just mentioned.

Ali adapted both at work and socially by learning to remain quiet. She realized that she was losing her cognitive abilities but retained the presence of mind to be frightened about this fact, which she hid from others. Rather than engaging people as she normally would, she became a quiet spectator.

Finally, she stopped going to work and going out socially. Previously, Ali had used exercise for clarity of mind, but exercise no longer helped her get through the day. In the gym, she had become a danger to herself, tripping and falling on the treadmill and losing her grip on weights.

One day in early 2017, Ali left her neurologist's office with no hope of stopping the decline. She worried that she would not be there for her daughter. She sought evaluation for HSCT. Both Ali and her mother were told the possible risks, including mortality. For MS, the most significant risk for mortality with the nonmyeloablative regimen that I use and in a patient with no other comorbid disease is infection. Ali's mother began crying. Upon returning home, their neurologist, whom they trusted, told them, "You might die from HSCT, but right now you are dying a little each day." That made their decision.

Within three months after HSCT, Ali started working out and in time was able to do all the things she had stopped doing before HSCT. Today, three and a half years later, Ali is living a normal life. She is on no medications and has a normal memory. In Ali's words, "I am now living life on my terms." Her MS and recovery from it affected her philosophy of life. After a twenty-plus-year career, she left corporate America to become a health and life coach in order to help others. She says, "I am happier and healthier [now] than in the last twenty years." Ali renewed old friendships, and some friends gave her the nickname "ALI STRONG," which is now etched on her car's license plate.

Efficacy of HSCT on Neurologic Disability, Quality of Life, and Costs

The efficacy of HSCT depends on patient selection (select patients with relapsing-remitting MS and ongoing recent active relapses) and the treatment conditioning regimen (a nonmyeloablative, less toxic regimen is safer). Done right, the responses may be, for a given individual patient, astounding. To this day, medicine follows the established paradigm of chronic MS drugs to slow disease progression while implying that HSCT is some frivolous, hand-waving hocus-pocus. Developing this field, being at the bedside of each and every patient, being available 24/7, seeing these miracles daily, one must ask themselves, *Who is really living in a delusion?*

We reported the results of the randomized trial in the *Journal of the American Medical Association* in 2019. For active relapsing-remitting MS that was already failing MS drugs, HSCT improved neurologic disability. In comparison, neurologic disability worsened with continued MS drugs. After HSCT, quality of life improved because neurologic disability improved, and the patients stopped using MS drugs. Quality of life did not improve for patients who continued MS drugs because neurologic disability did not improve and patients stayed on chronic drugs with their inconveniences, side effects, and costs.

To illustrate differences in quality of life, Table 1 shows quality of life after HSCT (using our nonmyeloablative regimen) versus what has been reported in trials of FDA-approved MS drugs. As previously mentioned, the SF-36 is a standard quality of life questionnaire. It goes from 0 to 100 (the higher the number, the better one's quality of life). Again, most MS drug trials do not even report quality of life. The newest and strongest anti-MS drugs alemtuzumab (Lemtrada), natalizumab (Tysabri), and ocrelizumab (Ocrevus) did report quality of life (Table 1), but the changes were clinically meaningless; that is, the change was below the threshold that a patient would recognize as improvement.

Some have argued that these newer drugs did improve quality of life because, as they correctly point out, the quality of life improved in these drug studies by 0 to 2 points (on a scale of 0 to 100). However, the minimal change required for a patient to perceive an improvement in their life is an increase of 5 or more. That is, for a patient, the minimal change in SF-36 to appreciate an effect on quality of life is 5 points. As Shree and other patients have told me, their doctors call no new brain lesions an improvement. But what is important for the patient is their quality of life, freedom from the severe fatigue, loss of balance, urinary frequency/incontinence, weakness, numbness, mental fog, and other MS symptoms.

MS usually does not kill you. It robs you of who you are. It takes away the meaning and quality of life. What is the purpose of life if there is no quality and only continued worsening and suffering? What is critical for an MS patient is quality of life, especially returning to normal. And what is quality of life when on continued MS drugs, despite their chronic expense and side effects, your disease continues to worsen, slowed but unabated? There is a difference between statistical improvement in the numbers and clinical improvement for a patient. In comparison, quality of life improved by a clinically meaningful 15 to 25 points after nonmyeloablative HSCT (Table 1).

To further obscure comparison, the SF-36 has a physical component (PCS), a mental component (MCS), and a total score (physical plus mental). The few drug studies that reported quality of life usually did not report all three components (Table 1). After HSCT we report all three components: physical, (PCS), mental (MCS), and total score (Table 1).

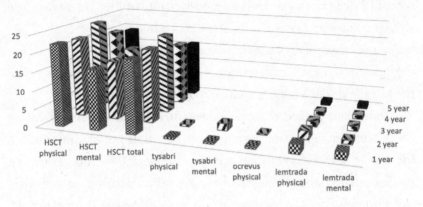

Table 1. Improvement in SF-36 quality of life (physical, mental, total) for relapsing-remitting multiple sclerosis for each year after nonmyeloablative hematopoietic stem cell transplant (HSCT) versus after drugs (Tysabri, Ocrevus, or Lemtrada). To be clinically meaningful, the improvement must be 5 or greater. (Tysabri is also called natalizumab; Ocrevus is also called ocrelizumab; Lemtrada or Campath is also called alemtuzumab.)

The charges for a transplant can fluctuate considerably, depending upon the regimen used and local variability. Myeloablative regimens are considerably more expensive, but when doing our nonmyeloablative regimen, the charges, as published in 2020, have remained stable at approximately $100,000. (Caveat emptor: a myeloablative regimen would be considerably more expensive.) This is a lot of money, whether paid for by a patient, insurance, or society. Almost all charges are hospital charges. (In the future, an even safer regimen done as an outpatient would be cheaper.) But what are the costs when compared to MS drugs?

MS drugs (DMTs) may be taken by swallowing a pill (oral) (Gilenya, Tecfidera, Mavenclad, Zeposia, Bafiertam, Aubagio, Mayzent, Vumerity, dimethyl fumerate); by infusion into a vein (intravenous) (Tysabri, Lemtrada, Ocrevus); or administered as an injection under the skin (subcutaneous) such as interferons (Betaseron, Rebif, Plegridy, Avonex, Extavia, Kesimpta), or glatiramer acetate (Copaxone, Glatopa, Mylan). Compared to the 1990s, when only interferons were available, this array of MS drugs is now a part of an impressive drug arsenal available against MS. They are, however, all based on suppressing the immune system, unlike HSCT, which is based on a one-time immune reset that utilizes a short course (five days) of usually patent-expired medications.

Each year, the cost of MS drugs has increased at a rate well above inflation and independent of the drug at identical hyperbolic rates, as if somehow invisibly tied to one another (Table 2). Should we believe, as Albert Einstein said about quantum mechanics, that this is some sort of "spooky action at a distance"? The interferons, when they first received FDA approval in the 1990s, cost around $9,000 a year. By 2020, they cost around $90,000 a year.[16][17] The interferons increased in price at the same accelerating trajectory as each newer, more expensive MS drug was approved and introduced to the market.

A patent is a government-sanctioned monopoly that is guaranteed for the life of the patent. The cost of the MS drug Copaxone precipitously decreased by more than 50 percent after losing patent protection.[18] The new, lower price may more accurately reflect today's profit after manufacturing and distribution costs.

This should not be construed as criticism directed toward patents or toward pharmaceutical companies, per se. Patents and protected licenses are appropriately designed to encourage investment and a return to society from that investment. Pharmaceutical companies endure tremendous obstacles involving overhead, risk, red tape, and bureaucracy, and are far too often made the scapegoat for societal ills. Rather, this should be viewed as a systemic problem arising from within the entire medical structure.

The reason for high drug costs is complex and goes beyond this book. But one contributing cause is extensive regulation. As Alexander Hamilton, whose picture is on the American ten dollar bill, said: "The passion of man will not conform to the dictates of reason and justice without constraints (regulations)." The irony within this logical statement is that unconstrained regulation, as a man-made

Generic name	Brand name	Year released	Approximate annual cost when released on market	Approximate 2020 annual cost
Interferon-beta 1b	Betaseron	1993	$19,000	$103,000
Interferon-beta 1a	Avenox	1996	$13,000	$92,000
Glatiramer acetate	Copaxone	1996	$12,000	$86,000
Interferon beta 1a	Rebif	2002	$20,000	$103,000
Natalizumab	Tysabri	2006	$31,000	$89,000
Interferon beta-1b	Extavia	2009	$35,000	$81,000
Fingolimod	Gilenya	2010	$56,000	$105,000
Teriflunomide	Aubagio	2012	$50,000	$93,000
Dimethyl fumarate	Tecfidera	2013	$60,000	$100,000
Peginterferon beta-1a	Plegridy	2014	$67,000	$92,000
Alemtuzumab	Lemtrada	2014	$71,000	$80,000
Ocrelizumab	Ocrevus	2017	$68,000	$65,000
Siponimod	Mayzent	2019	$89,000	$93,000
Cladribine	Mavenclad	2019	$100,000	$107,000
Diroximel fumarate	Vumerity	2019	$88,000	$88,000

Table 2. Yearly Cost of MS drugs

construct, is itself susceptible to the unreasonable and unjust consequences of man's fervor. If you doubt the contribution of regulations to drug costs, try reading Title 21 of the Code of Federal Regulations (CFR) or the International Council for Harmonization (ICH). The CFR and ICH provide technical requirements for pharmaceutical trials. These regulations have continuously expanded over the decades and are extensive, complex, written to rigid minutiae, and expensive to implement, monitor, and document compliance.

Ten of the last eleven FDA commissioners became members of pharmaceutical companies after leaving the FDA. This is not a criticism of any of these distinguished individuals but a statement of a reality that arises naturally from our current medical system. Because no one else has the expertise with complex FDA regulations, a revolving door has developed that in practicality needs to exist between pharmaceutical companies and the FDA (Table 3). It has become an expensive game that very few can afford to play but one in which patients and society pay the costs.

While the FDA regulates drug (and/or device) production and licensing, the FDA currently does not—and should not—regulate the bedside practice of medicine. The practice of medicine is regulated by physicians and other medical professionals after decades of selection, training, testing, documentation of expertise, and certification of these qualifications via licensing.

Compared to MS drugs, HSCT is only performed once, after which most patients remain drug-free for more than five years and perhaps, as described herein, two or more decades. One year of paying for MS drugs would pay for the entire transplant when using a nonmyeloablative regimen (as a buyer-beware caveat, myeloablative regimens are far more expensive). When a patient's job is terminated, they lose their insurance and can no longer afford such expensive MS drugs, as Eretria's story so powerfully exposes. When that happens, patients often go untreated. In contrast, after HSCT, independent of employment or insurance status, most no longer need MS drugs.

As the psychiatrist Jenny mused in her story about perceptions and preconceived bias, are the real money profiters doing HSCT in some back alley or is the problem within our own medical structure? Reiterating a twist from naval officer Oliver Perry's famous quote from the War of 1812, perhaps, "We have met the enemy, and he is us."

FDA commissioner	Years as head of FDA	Position after FDA	Pharmaceutical company
Arthur Hayes	1981–1983	President	E.M. Pharmaceuticals
Frank Young	1984–1989	Vice President	Braeburn Pharmaceuticals
Jane Henney	1999–2001	Member of the Board	Amerisource-Bergen and AstraZeneca
Mark McClellan	2002–2004	Member of the Board	Johnson & Johnson
Lester Crawford	2005–2005	Member of the Board	Bexion Pharmaceuticals
Andrew von Eschenback	2006–2009	Member of the Board	Bausch Health Inc. and Viamet Pharmaceuticals
Margaret Hamburg	2009–2015	Member of the Board	Alnylam Pharmaceuticals
Robert Califf	2016–2017	Senior Advisor	Verily
Scott Gottlieb	2017–2019	Member of the Board	Pfizer Inc.
Stephen Hahn	2019–2021	Chief Medical Officer and Partner	Flagship Pioneering (Moderna) and Harbinger Health

Table 3. FDA commissioners who subsequently joined pharmaceutical companies

New Nonmyeloablative Regimens

The complication of ITP is relatively (but not entirely) specific for MS and for particular conditioning regimens. HSCT using a nonmyeloablative regimen of Cytoxan and ATG worked phenomenally well. The risk of ITP (sudden drop in platelets that clot blood) occurred in only 2 percent of HSCT patients, compared to Cytoxan and alemtuzumab, where it occurred in about 12 percent. While it is readily reversed if treated, my worry is that a patient would ignore warning symptoms of easy or spontaneous bruising. I wanted to completely eliminate the risk of ITP with a new nonmyeloablative regimen. I wrote new protocols and tried two different nonmyeloablative conditioning regimens: Cytoxan/ATG/IVIG (intravenous immunoglobulins), or, for more aggressive cases of MS, Cytoxan/ATG/Rituxan (rituximab).

HSCT 4 MS

Anna is a medical professional. Her children could not remember their mother without MS. She was in the hospital, between patients, and writing a note when without warning and without pain, her right eye "whited out." It was as if that eye had been covered by bright white paper. The rest of the day, she continued working, doing her duty for her patients and never letting on what was happening to her. Over a two-week interval, she saw an optician, an optometrist, an ophthalmologist, and finally a neuro-ophthalmologist. She was told that she had optic neuritis (inflammation of an eye nerve).

An MRI confirmed the diagnosis of MS. Anna started steroids and was told to take one month off from work. An MS drug (Copaxone) was prescribed by a Cleveland Clinic specialist. Anna kept working but also kept relapsing. Sick leave absences started piling up. Copaxone did not work. Her doctors prescribed another MS drug (an interferon called Avenox). Despite each injection making her feel horribly ill, she faithfully followed their medical advice. After each self-injection, Anna would become totally disabled for one or two days from the drug's side effects.

Her left arm no longer obeyed her conscious will. Instead of purposeful movement, it would involuntarily jerk. She had to start permanent disability. Her physical therapy was in the same department where she herself used to treat patients. A limp with foot drop developed. Her left foot would not bend up, as she had lost dorsiflexion.

Her parents, who lived in another state, left their home, their retirement, and their friends behind to come help Anna. They built a new home in a neighborhood a few blocks away and took on the daily care of their grandchildren. Anna's parents had already spent a lifetime raising their daughter. Without having to be asked, without financial assistance, and without hesitation, they accepted parenting responsibility for their grandsons and accepted the reparenting of their daughter.

Anna's doctors prescribed a third MS drug (Gilenya). This time the side effects were worse. She lost twenty-five pounds and had no appetite. Her heart started skipping beats and racing. At times her pulse ran so fast that she could not catch her breath. After four months on Gilenya, Anna was told by her cardiologist to immediately stop taking it and never take it again. Heart rhythm problems are a known major complication of Gilenya. Her doctors recommended a fourth MS drug.

Anna had lost confidence in MS medications. They were expensive, made her sick, did not stop relapses, and new brain lesions continued. This time, after the third MS drug strikeout, she rejected her doctors' advice. She needed a drug holiday. Anna changed her diet, started low-dose naltrexone, and underwent treatment with CCSVI (a term for treating narrow veins in the neck that some had suggested may be the cause for some types of MS). Nothing worked. By 2012, she was on long-term disability and could not drive at night or in the rain. Her parents had to drive her children to their after-school activities. Anna's life had become a permanent liability for her children, her husband, and her parents. She was drowning and dragging them down with her. One way or another, she knew this had to stop.

Cleveland Clinic collected mesenchymal stem cells (MSC) from Anna's hip and injected them into her veins. Six months later, she had another acute attack. She and about two dozen patients who were in the mesenchymal stem cell study were told that the treatment did not work. The trial was over. The MSC were well-tolerated but did not improve neurologic disability.[19]

As mentioned in chapter 3, there are many types of stem cells. Mesenchymal stem cells are not the same as hematopoietic stem cells. The isolation, technique, rationale, methods, results, indications, applications, and regulations for HSCT and mesenchymal stem cells are totally different. Mesenchymal stem cells are themselves highly variable. Depending upon the source (for example, placenta, fat, or bone marrow), culture conditions, passage number (number of times expanded in culture), biologic cell age (age of the donor), whether allogenic (from another person) or autologous (from your own body), and the site of administration (injected into a vein or injected into a tissue), the results from mesenchymal stem cells could be different.

Similarly, some people think that all autologous HSCTs for MS are the same. They are not. The toxicity and results of HSCT for MS and other autoimmune diseases depend upon the conditioning regimen used and patient selection.

Anna was started on a fourth MS drug called Tysabri. After three years of Tysabri, which Anna told me cost $12,000 a month, she developed a new MS brain lesion and was struggling with even worse fatigue, had more visual problems, and was using a cane and walker as well as a wheelchair for traveling longer distances. When the family went to Disney World, Anna had to be pushed in a wheelchair by her husband and mother-in-law. Doctors at Cleveland Clinic advised her to start a fifth MS drug called Lemtrada (also known as alemtuzumab). Despite the formal center recommendation, one of the younger Cleveland Clinic doctors pulled Anna aside and informally told her to get HSCT and where to go. This was the state of HSCT for MS—a young neurologist outside of the "official" hierarchy guided her toward HSCT.

Anna underwent HSCT using a regimen of Cytoxan, ATG, and Rituxan. Over the last three and a half years, she has taken no more drugs and has had no more attacks. She can walk without assistance. If she walks long distance, a limp will transiently return, but she does not need to use a cane or other device. Her vision recovered and she can now see and drive under all conditions, even at night. In fact, she is now the neighborhood driver for after-school events and extracurricular activities. Her parents returned to their out-of-state home and to their own lives. Anna is a mom, a wife, and a daughter again. Her children now know their mother without MS.

When I was writing this book, Anna and her husband told me that MS is an acronym for MonSter, and that every day they think about and are thankful for HSCT. She and her family recently returned from vacationing at Disneyland. There, Anna walked all day without assistance—no wheelchair, no walker, no cane. She exercises every day, and she sent me a picture of herself standing on her head while doing yoga. Her license plate reads "HSCT 4 MS."

Azza

Azza is a woman from the United Arab Emirates (UAE), a country in the Persian Gulf. She was married with a small child. She and her husband were planning to start a company together in the UAE when she was suddenly hit by MS. Her neurologists referred her to the Cleveland Clinic in the United States. She had only been diagnosed three months earlier and came to America walking without assistance.

After about three months in Cleveland, she was in a wheelchair and declining fast. Cleveland Clinic referred her to me for HSCT.

I was told to wait for the international office to arrange her transfer. After about five to six weeks of waiting and after speaking with one of her neurologists at Cleveland Clinic, I said to myself, *Forget this.* I was not going to wait for the bureaucracy of international offices from two hospitals to arrange a transfer that was being held up by a confirmation of money. I called the UAE embassy in Washington, DC, myself and reached their medical director. Understanding the urgency of the situation, he immediately reached out to his contacts in the UAE for approval. Azza was transferred to me within a few days.

When I came into her room, I was stunned. Azza was in a deep coma and had been like that for a week. A sternal rub (rubbing the chest plate between the ribs with your closed knuckles) elicited absolutely no response. My own spirits sank. Through an interpreter, I informed the family that HSCT may not help her and that we may be too late. The family went ballistic. I understood them, and I did not blame them. When she had come to America a few months earlier, she had been walking and had appeared normal. They were told that they were coming to America for the best treatment in the world. The family asked me not to give up, or at least to try my best.

Azza's MRI showed numerous lesions, including lesions in the brain stem (the central trunk of the brain that connects the higher brain to the spinal cord) that accounted for her deep coma. The only hopeful sign was that several lesions were enhancing, indicating ongoing inflammatory activity.

For the first time, I started HSCT on a comatose patient. In private, I thought that I had lost my mind. If things went badly, and I was asked to justify the transplant, I could not. As far as I knew, nobody had ever performed HSCT on a comatose patient for cancer or for any disease, nor would they. Was this a hopeless Hail Mary pass into the end zone after regular time had expired?

It is worth restating that the foundation of Western law and of my care for a patient rest upon their consent. Everything, even accepting the risks and side effects of either a prescription drug or an over-the-counter nonprescription drug, always comes back to consent. Your body, your life—your consent is needed. If a patient cannot speak for themselves, the next of kin provides the consent. In Azza's case, the husband, mother, and brother were in unanimous agreement.

If I tried and failed, other people would ridicule me, but I could live with that. I had been ridiculed for decades since I first had had the idea to perform HSCT for MS. But if I did not try, I would not be able to live with myself. I used the usual regimen of cyclophosphamide and ATG but added rituximab and IVIG. I would have thrown in the kitchen sink if I'd thought it would help. I also knew that when you commit to something no one else has ever done, like crossing the river Tiber, your own self-confidence will build confidence in others. When I was on the debate team in high school, I was always told to act with confidence, even when I was feeling uncertain.

Azza had walked into the clinic in Cleveland with the easy, flowing gait of someone still certain that the world was hers to experience. The family showed me videos of her in the UAE. She was confident, well-educated, and innately intelligent. It is said that the loose, flowing black *hijab* (head cover) and *niqab* (face cover) hide a woman's beauty, but it did not conceal Azza's beauty. Her pure, midnight-black eyes sparkled with life.

After HSCT, Azza awoke from her coma. At first, she could only manage to almost imperceptibly squeeze my hand until, with each passing day, she could eventually lift her arm. Every morning when I went on rounds, her mother, who spoke no English, would offer me fresh tea that she had just made when I entered Azza's room. I do not know how she did it, but it was and still is the best tea I have ever tasted.

After transplant, Azza needed extensive rehabilitation. A few months after returning home, the family emailed me a video of Azza walking outside without assistance. She only walked about twenty-five feet from a chair to the side of the house. She had to concentrate. It was effort. She forced her legs to move in small steps instead of taking effortless strides. She was unsteady, but she did it.

Five years post-transplant, Azza has had no MS medications or new attacks. HSCT brought her back, but not all the way. She still needs a wheelchair. If HSCT for MS had been more available or if she had gotten to me a few weeks earlier, she probably would have made it all the way back.

By culture and custom, Azza always covered her head and face, but when she was around me, whether in the hospital or clinic, she would remove her face and head covers. I realized that she did this out of respect for me. She knew I was from a different culture and wanted to make me feel comfortable. I have always been impressed by how my patients show concern for me and want me to be comfortable. For others, Azza always kept her head and face covered. Either way, I could see her dark Arabian eyes—midnight-black eyes that sparkled like the stars of the Milky Way in the middle of a desert night.

Five years after her HSCT, I was invited to teach at a conference in Abu Dhabi. Azza lived in a different emirate of the United Arab Emirates. I asked if I could see her. I offered to meet her in Ras Al Khaimah, but again she insisted on my convenience. She came to Abu Dhabi, a three-hour drive from her home, to see me.

She was in a wheelchair but could walk a short distance with difficulty. She could dress and care for herself, and she was a mother to her young son. Azza's dream of starting her own company had been killed by MS, but despite residual atrophy and damage, she had taught herself English and understood every word I said.

Her brother, dressed in a traditional dishdasha (white garment), had accompanied her. A powerfully built man, he reminded me of an Arabian knight from an earlier epoch. Like Santiago in *The Alchemist* by Brazilian author Paulo Coelho, I had performed an honorable act for his sister. In his eyes, in Azza's eyes, and by Arab tradition and culture, they would now always protect me.

I had helped Azza but not nearly enough. HSCT resets the immune system, but the hematopoietic stem cell does not itself repair damaged tissue. For ten years now, I have tested in animals a new, very early (pluripotent) stem cell that can repair damaged organs. With these genetically modified pluripotent cells, I have returned to where I was decades ago before starting HSCT. There are no guarantees that it will work in humans, but if it does (Inshallah), I will not forget Azza nor any of my patients.

Patient Support Groups

In the Internet age, patients undergoing HSCT for MS (and other autoimmune diseases) often find one another through social media. When official societies and channels are not supportive, as has been the experience for HSCT, patients set up their own support systems. Online support sites, including Facebook groups, take significant time from at least one or more patients to organize, manage, and maintain. All of this is done without resources, recognition, or personal reimbursement.

Facebook support sites include patient social events, comments, and shared patient experiences. It is completely appropriate and often helpful for patients to join these online communities. However, medical professionals are trained never to communicate or release information about any patient (without prior written permission) or to post on any unvetted site.

We are taught as physicians that information can be used to destroy people as ruthlessly as any crime. Rape is an act performed for the twisted psychological pleasure of humiliating another person. Words can be a form of psychological rape that give the perp the same perverse distorted—but legal—psychological pleasure.

I am not on social media, but most of my staff are. I always convey to my staff not to enter these patient support sites. To do so would be like putting listening devices in a patient waiting room. No sane professional could or should do such a thing. I view patient online and social media communication, including Facebook, as privileged patient-to-patient communication.

In America, the National MS Society has, for the longest time, at best ignored HSCT, and I fear it still does not appreciate the difference between nonmyeloablative and myeloablative conditioning regimens. Some patients bridged this vacuum by organizing other nonprofits and/or educational events. Failure of standard organizations is the impetus for innovative healthcare solutions. What I have long known is that every problem also generates an opportunity. Seize the opportunity.

Sleeping Beauty and AIMS

Having had three children while in her twenties and becoming a single mother, Shari was consumed with her children and her work. Since about twenty-five years of age, she'd had one thing on her bucket list—to run a marathon. The pressures of everyday life kept pushing her marathon wish off into the "next year," but she was still determined to run one.

Her MS symptoms started a few years before diagnosis. The first symptom was an electric shock running down her spine (Lhermitte's sign) when trying to touch her neck with her chin (neck flexion). Lhermitte's sign would come and go intermittently over two years. Numbness in her left hand or arm would also come and go. Her doctors told her that as a single mom, she was under stress and had to get rest. One doctor prescribed an antidepressant. She insisted that she was not depressed but relented to medical advice and started taking the antidepressant drug. Paradoxically, one side effect of antidepressants is depression and suicidal ideation (thoughts). The antidepressant did nothing at all to help her symptoms.

Shari remarried and traveled to Italy for her honeymoon. During her honeymoon, something went wrong. Her body went into hibernation. She was exhausted and kept falling asleep throughout the day. While her husband was standing at the train station looking for the next scheduled train on the overhead sign, she sat down on the luggage, slumped against the wall, and in the middle of the day fell asleep. Her husband was carrying Sleeping Beauty across Italy. When dealing with MS, the kiss of a prince cannot break the spell.

Upon returning to America, Shari developed visual problems (optic neuritis) and the left side of her face began to sag. Her mouth turned down in a frown on the left while the right side turned up in a smile. At the age of thirty-six, she was diagnosed with MS.

While taking the MS drug Avenox, she became nauseated. Some blood tests were ordered. The doctor's office called her and told her to immediately stop taking Avenox because it was damaging her liver. After recovering from liver injury, she started another MS drug, Copaxone, but it had no effect. She kept relapsing. She had been on high doses of steroids for eighteen months that caused her to gain one hundred pounds. Weight gain is one of a legion of side effects from steroids. The steroids also caused avascular necrosis (death of bone tissue due to lack of blood supply) of her knee joints that was treated after HSCT with injection of stem cells (probably mesenchymal stem cells) with resolution of joint pain. After eighteen months of high-dose steroids, her pharmacist refused to continue filling physician-written steroid prescriptions.

Shari worked as a paralegal, but her memory was becoming so bad that she had to write everything down or she would forget. She developed bilateral foot drop and was ordered AFOs (ankle braces) and a walker. She never filled the order. Instead, she started using bilateral walking sticks. Her left hand jerked involuntarily.

She remembered that early after her diagnosis, she had spoken with a gentleman at a Halloween party who told her that his sister had MS and has remained free of MS symptoms for ten years after receiving HSCT. Shari thought how upside down the world could be that her specialist doctors did not know about nor could recommend a transplant. Instead, she learned about it from a nonmedical professional, a neighbor.

While lying in the hospital bed going through transplant, Shari reflected upon how she had missed doing the one thing that was on her bucket list—running a marathon. She had put it off, and now she no longer had that option. She was simply hoping that HSCT would arrest her MS so she would not get any worse as she did not think she would get better. She did not improve right away. It was one year before she was able to get rid of her canes. It was three years before she could start running and training for a marathon, but Shari achieved her goal. She ran her first marathon in the city of her transplant. She completed it and gave me her bib that she had worn during the race.

In 2021, she ran a trifecta of marathons within three weeks: London, Berlin, and Boston. She had met the BQ (Boston-qualifying) time a year earlier. Shari ran the London marathon to raise money for the Auto Immune and Multiple Sclerosis (AIMS) charity.[20]

Life is interconnected and full of coincidences. Undergoing HSCT for MS connected Shari to AIMS on the opposite side of the Atlantic Ocean. AIMS was started by Alison and her husband, James, about one year after James's transplant for MS in the United Kingdom. Alison advertised on social media requesting a volunteer to run the London Marathon to help raise money for the AIMS charity. Shari, who lived in America, responded. She was a godsend because she *herself* had undergone HSCT for MS. Alison and Shari became fast friends. The London Marathon organizers allocated AIMS a charity entry, and Shari completed the race in October 2021.

Alison, the founder of AIMS, has taught speech, theater, debate, communication, and presentation skills. She is a natural at recognizing communications barriers. She told me that the barriers to HSCT in the UK (and US) are lack of practitioners able to carry out HSCT for MS; lack of medical centers providing HSCT for MS; lack of education among transplant hematologists about MS; lack of education among neurologists about HSCT; a reluctance by neurologists to refer patients; and a failure to understand that the toxicity and efficacy depend on the conditioning regimen used for the transplant.

HSCT tied Shari, Allison, and AIMS together for the purpose of helping people understand and get HSCT.

HSCT Hope

During her first year of law school on the day before her twenty-third birthday, Cassidy was diagnosed with relapsing-remitting multiple sclerosis. She was prescribed and remained on the MS drug Rebif, which was injected into her every Monday, Wednesday, and Friday for the duration of law school. Because the injections caused severe, flulike muscle aches, she scheduled her Tuesday and Thursday law classes for late afternoons or evenings. Due to the muscle aches (myalgia), Cassidy could not function in the morning after the previous day's injection. Even by afternoon, she had to wear body-hugging stockings under which she hid hot packs to help offset drug-induced muscle pain while she was sitting in the classroom.

Due to severe MS-related fatigue and mental fog, Cassidy took various stimulants sequentially (Ritalin, Adderall, Provigil, Nuvigil). When one stimulant became ineffective, she traded it for another. Law school is difficult enough for healthy people. Despite muscle aches, fatigue, and mental fog, Cassidy fought on and graduated on time.

On her first day of work at the law firm where she had been hired, she found out about a case that was before the state supreme court.

When she learned that it involved a woman in her fifties who had MS and was in a nursing home, her stomach dropped.

After a severe acute relapse, her MS drug was changed to Tysabri, the most potent drug available at the time. Eventually, Cassidy started her own boutique law firm with her own support staff to help handle the case volume. After eighteen months and a sudden flare of MS-triggered vertigo (room and walls spinning) that caused her to collapse, stumble like a drunk, and run into courthouse walls, she hired an associate attorney to join her practice to help her manage cases. Due to continued relapses and testing positive for JC virus, Cassidy stopped taking Tysabri. Within two months of starting her third MS drug, Copaxone, she relapsed again. Copaxone was replaced with her fourth MS drug, Tecfidera, that had just arrived on the market.

While on Tecfidera, Cassidy could not eat and kept a garbage can next to her office desk for the sudden episodes of vomiting that were a Tecfidera side effect. After three months, she had lost twenty pounds. Tecfidera was replaced by Gilenya, her fifth MS drug. It caused suicidal thoughts (a known side effect). At this point, she tried to save her practice by partnering with another law firm. In the end, she had to go on disability and gave up practicing law altogether. MS had fought to prevent her from becoming a lawyer, and after eleven years, it finally won. Her legal career was finished.

Cassidy's HSCT was uncomplicated, but neurologic improvement was slower than most patients perhaps due to her fifteen-year-long history with MS. Fatigue and insomnia did not improve until more than one year later. Since her HSCT treatment over three years ago, Cassidy has been free of MS drugs and has been able to discontinue high doses of a pain drug (gabapentin), stop taking a mood stabilizer, significantly cut back on the sleeping pills that she had needed for pre-HSCT MS-related insomnia, and stop urinary incontinence medication. Her MS mental fog has completely lifted.

Cassidy now runs her own legal consulting company. She offers legal writing and coaching for attorneys and firms and is starting a nonprofit, HSCT Hope, to help patients fight insurance companies and write GoFundMe pages in order to get HSCT.

Warrior

Julie was a twenty-nine-year-old lawyer with her own practice when she began having headaches, sometimes so severe that it felt like her head would explode. She was diagnosed with migraines. A few months later, she awoke with some numbness on her left side. Her work and commitment to her clients took priority, so she ignored the numbness, treating it like a mild nuisance, anticipating that it would go away.

Later that morning, while riding as a passenger in a car, the road blurred in front of her. She felt drunk, but it was only 8:00 a.m. and she was stone-cold sober. As the day progressed, she became exhausted, as if all her batteries had suddenly been drained dry. The urge to sleep was overwhelming. Julie convinced a friend to drive her back home at noon. As soon as she entered her apartment, she collapsed on her bed and did not wake up until the next day, eighteen hours later.

When she woke up the numbness had spread farther across her body. Julie knew she needed to see a doctor, but instead she jumped in her car to get to work. Whatever was going on, her obligations to others came first. Two blocks from her house, her vision blurred again. She could not tell if oncoming cars were parked on the street or if they were accelerating down the road toward her. She abandoned her car and walked to the train station to get to work.

When Julie arrived in the lobby of her law office, a coworker asked her if she had hurt her leg over the weekend. She queried why she would ask. Her coworker looked inquiringly toward Julie and said, "You are limping." Julie had no idea she had a limp until that moment.

Julie still had to appear in court that morning. She limped the few blocks' walk from her office to the courthouse. By the time the case was called, she could not read the papers in her hand. Words started running together. She limped and careened from one wall to the next while heading back to her office. Crossing the street was the most dangerous part. Only by covering one eye could she identify from which direction the traffic was coming.

When she got home, Julie called her mother, a nurse, who insisted on an emergency appointment with an eye doctor. The ophthalmologist found nothing wrong with Julie's eyes and told her she needed to head to the ER immediately. After hours in the emergency room waiting area, she went from limping to being unable to walk. She had to be wheeled into the ER exam room to be evaluated. The doctor immediately ordered a brain scan (MRI) as Julie had become completely blind in one eye, was unable to walk, and could barely stand.

Her mother and the neurologist walked together into her ER room to discuss the MRI results. She had MS—her MRI of the brain lit up like a Christmas tree with lesions too numerous to count. Looking through the one eye that still had vision, Julie saw tears streaming down her mother's face. She knew she was in trouble. From that time forward, her life as she knew it was over.

MS hit her like a freight train but then played with her like a cat with a mouse. She got better on steroids, returned to 90 percent functionality, hoped she would not have to deal with MS again for some time, tried to keep her law office open, and even started planning her wedding.

Within a few months, Julie awoke with one side of her body and face again feeling numb and asleep. She could not slap it awake. Dysarthria (slurred mumbling words) and aphasia (unable to find the words) set in. She found herself back in the hospital, getting steroids and starting on a chronic MS drug. MS was now dictating her life decisions. She was no longer in control of her body. She had to surrender the dream of her own law practice.

Six weeks later Julie was again back in the hospital with her third relapse and received even more steroids. This time she had lost control of movement in her left arm and hand. After three relapses in six months, her MS drug was switched to Tysabri. Tysabri was infused into her veins once a month and caused a slew of new side effects, but it was the best anti-MS drug available.

Life on Tysabri allowed her to work part time as a member of another law firm, but fatigue was constant. If she worked a full day, she needed to take the next day off to sleep. Or she could work in the morning but then needed to go home in the afternoon to sleep for several hours before dinner. Julie could never go out on a Friday night. She was too exhausted. She could go out for dinner on Saturday night, but only by first sleeping for several hours in the afternoon.

Two years after diagnosis, Julie underwent transplant using a regimen of cyclophosphamide, ATG, and IVIG. After transplant, she got her life back. Ninety-nine percent of her MS symptoms have gone away. She experiences zero numbness, her vision is normal (a perfect 20/20 visual acuity), and she has remained drug-free. To celebrate her one-year HSCT birthday, she decided to do something that had always been on her bucket list. She bought a car, packed up her dog, and took a cross-country road trip. Post-transplant, she has even traveled to Europe twice and walked forty-eight miles over the course of a week-long vacation at Disney World. Most important for Julie, she returned to practicing law full time and reopened her own practice.

Her first MS neurologist had told her that she would be wheelchair-bound by the age of thirty-five. During the writing of this book, Julie turned thirty-five. She is living a normal life. She told me, "There is no wheelchair in sight and no MS drugs are on the horizon for me!"

Julie fought MS like a warrior and after HSCT, she, along with other patients who underwent HSCT for MS, helped found an online resource called HSCT Warriors (https://www.facebook.com /hsctwarriors).

Podcast

While in the hospital going through HSCT, another of my patients, Jen, realized that starting a podcast could help other MS patients. She launched the HSCT Warriors podcast (https://hsctwarriorspodcast .com/) to connect with other people through shared experiences and education, to help other patients, and to break down locked and rigid mental concepts.

There is space in this book to mention only the efforts of a few patients who have tried to educate and help other people suffering from MS and other diseases. As mentioned, there are multiple Facebook and social media sites, but since I do not follow social media, I do not know of most of them. Nevertheless, I recognize that patients who have established social media sites are trying without reimbursement or solicitation of funds to educate people just as hard as the patients mentioned herein are voluntarily doing. These patients are the living embodiment of altruism. They give selflessly of their time and expertise for the well-being and education of others.

Insurance Approval

If a patient appeared to be a candidate, I and my nurse would submit documentation for insurance approval. This takes a lot of time and work, but I would do this gratis. I would summarize the patient's medical history, state of the art in the field, and quote and attach my own and other publications. Then I would wait. Medicaid used to pay for HSCT, but after the Affordable Care Act (ACA) everything changed. The answer was always *no*, and there was never anyone who would speak with me.

Private insurance companies would sometimes approve with the first submission. Other times they denied coverage, and I would speak to the medical director. Sometimes the medical director would overturn the denial. Other times they would just say that they had no authority in the decision, mostly in a polite and appropriate manner.

The final step was the appeals process, which for private insurance usually went through a committee. I would usually, but not always, win on appeal. Because I had started it, I knew the field like the back of my hand, so presenting a case and answering questions was easy. I would love when they allowed the patient to be in on a phone conference; we would tag-team them.

The key is to speak to someone who has authority and wants to hear the patient's story and your information. Medicine has become so complex and specialized that no one could or would know or be appropriately informed and updated on information without these presentations. It is important to have someone to talk to, because inevitably, the appeal letter and all the publications supporting HSCT for MS that I would attach with the original submission or with each appeal never made into the hands of any of the committee members. Not even one time. Not even to appeal committees. When I asked the committee if they had received or read the information we had sent, the response was silence. But we always kept sending and offering to resend the paperwork justifying the treatment.

Litigation

University classes are difficult enough for anyone. Jen had to work double shifts as a waitress and bartender to pay for her education while getting a double major. She graduated with honors with a doctorate in education. In 2009, while at Northern Kentucky University, her hand suddenly went numb. In 2010, a day after being diagnosed with MS, she learned that she was pregnant with her first child.

What bad luck had befallen her, to be diagnosed with MS and pregnant at the same time. She knew what MS could do to her, but she worried for her child more than for herself. She could not predict the future or who would be there for her child. But in the here and now, she could refuse any MS drugs that may affect her unborn baby and cause developmental abnormalities. When faced with a choice to protect herself or her child, there was never any doubt, never any real choice. Jen chose to protect her baby and refused the MS drugs.

By grace or good fortune, pregnancy put Jen into a clinical remission. She practiced yoga and took her child hiking and rock climbing with her. With her child and a backpack, she would "cruise through the woods." In 2013, on her neurologist's recommendation, she began an MS drug. The morning of starting a five-mile hike through Red River Gorge, she took Tecfidera. A week later, her MS exploded. After that attack, she could never again hike or stand on her toes or even walk for twenty-five minutes on a treadmill. She was switched to Tysabri. Tysabri did not work, and new lesions continued to appear. Jen underwent a second workup to look for anything else besides MS that might be wrong. She was then diagnosed with both MS and Lyme disease. No matter what her doctors tried, she continued to get worse.

One day Jen picked up a Northern Kentucky University magazine. By chance it fell open to an article about a student with MS who had gotten a hematopoietic stem cell transplant.

Despite insurance bills of over $4,000 every month for drugs that were not stopping her MS, her insurance company would not pay for the transplant. In her case, the insurance company played a particularly wicked game. It sent her a letter that HSCT had been approved and then followed up with another letter of denial. For six months, she tried to appeal, but the door was closed. Nobody at the insurance company was listening to her. And the hospital would not allow HSCT without insurance approval or a monetary payment. During the eighteen months of insurance delay, she started to transition toward secondary progressive MS. At this point, Jen's family came through with a deposit. All members of her family sacrificed to help; her parents even sold their house to raise money for her treatment.

It has been four years since HSCT. Jen has remained drug-free. Her symptoms of numbness, tingling, and falling have resolved. Her balance is now normal, with no more wavering or staggering. Her left arm is more mobile, and she can bend her left knee that had previously been locked straight. Tremors in her legs resolved. Jen can stand on her toes and walk for twenty-five minutes on a treadmill, neither of which she could do for several years before HSCT. She continues to see slow improvements every year but cannot yet hike her favorite trail, Cloud Splitter.

After the transplant, Jen filed litigation against the insurance company and settled through mediation in order to reimburse her family who had paid for the transplant. Jen did not get any money for herself. She only asked for and received enough compensation to cover her family's financial expense.

Standing by Your Patients in Disease

Ivy was captain of her high school soccer team, president of the student honor society and prom queen. She was intelligent, beautiful, and well-liked. Her outgoing, friendly personality put everyone at ease, including me. Having been accepted into the university of her choice, Brigham Young University (BYU), her life was moving in the right direction. The only harbinger of a foreboding future was that, since age sixteen, she would intermittently develop numbness on one or another side of her body. When she looked down, electric-like pain shot from the bottom of her spine up her back and into the base of her skull. The symptoms would resolve within one to two weeks and were attributed to growing pains or a pinched nerve.

At age twenty, while watching *Mary Poppins*, she suddenly developed painless double vision (diplopia). At the local hospital emergency room where her father was a staff physician, Ivy was diagnosed with multiple sclerosis. She was stunned. A family friend had also just been diagnosed with MS. Ivy was young and carefree, and she never thought that three months later, she also would have MS. She started to cry. Her father was worried, but he put on a brave face. He embraced her and reassured her, "Do not worry. There is so much we can do." After receiving intravenous steroids, she left the emergency room wearing an eye patch.

As a trained ER physician, Ivy's father searched the medical literature and found and read our randomized *JAMA* trial. A neurologist had already recommended starting Tysabri due to Ivy's lesion load on MRI. Since HSCT requires a five-month Tysabri washout, her father had hoped she would get HSCT instead of Tysabri. He did not tell Ivy about HSCT until after we agreed to evaluate her. As a father, he wanted to protect her from false hope, just in case we declined to see her.

Hair regrows, but during HSCT, the patient will temporarily lose the hair on their head. Ivy's seventeen-year-old sister shaved her head as a sign of psychological support. Her father also volunteered to shave his head. Out of love and concern for her father and with a hug and a kiss, Ivy told him, "I must own this myself." I have been repeatedly amazed by the courage of my patients.

Before MS, Ivy was taking a crazy load of sixteen credits a semester, which she had dropped to nine credits when MS started. After HSCT, she took a normal load of twelve credits per semester. She felt fully capable of returning to sixteen credits, but because of MS and now a second chance at life, she wanted to graduate on time instead of early. This second time around, she took time to share her college experience with her lucky boyfriend.

After HSCT, Ivy volunteered for an internship with the MS Society and acted as a communication and content director for a local chapter. She kept pushing them to recognize and inform patients about HSCT. While the United Kingdom MS society (MS Society UK) was an advocate for HSCT from the get-go, for decades the US National MS Society had remained skeptical or, at best, just silent.

Since HSCT, Ivy has become a certified yoga instructor, hikes every summer, and skis in Park City every winter. She just accepted a job offer, but first she and her sister, who had shaved her head in support of Ivy's transplant, are going on a BYU-sponsored study abroad. They will be traveling to the Blue Zones (longevity hotspots) of Italy and Greece, home to the world's longest-living men and woman and largest concentration of centenarians. Ivy no longer wears her "pirate eye" patch.

Ivy's father paid for the transplant. Their insurance company refused. He is a physician himself, and a randomized trial had already demonstrated HSCT to be superior to the best MS drugs available, but it did not matter to the insurance provider. With each of his appeals, they declared that HSCT was experimental or medically unnecessary. Ivy told them, "Look at your motto: 'Standing by our patients in health.' Well, what about standing by your patients in disease? What about me? Patients do not need help during health. You're not standing by me when I have disease. You are not standing by me during my need." Her words were not heard.

I had previously interacted with this company's medical director, who was particularly intransient. Before that person was promoted to medical director, the company's prior medical director for over a decade always approved HSCT for MS. Do not ask names; it is unethical for me to provide them without permission, but as I recall, this insurance company had also approved HSCT for MS for one of its corporate executive's relatives. It is a large medical insurer. Most likely, the right hand did not know what the left hand was doing.

Double Whammy

Patrick was diagnosed with type 1 diabetes when he was eight years old. While others his age played games, diabetes instilled an early and strict discipline and routine in Patrick's life: regimented diet, regular insulin injections, repeated monitoring of blood sugar, and different insulin doses at different times of day with respect to changes in meals or activities. Despite good control of his hemoglobin A1C (a measure of chronic blood sugar levels), which diminished the risk of late complications, he developed diabetic-induced peripheral neuropathy. Diabetes damaged the nerves that ran from his spinal cord to his muscles. In 2009, another chronic disease that damaged his brain and spinal cord, relapsing-remitting MS, entered his life. Over time, he was prescribed three different MS drugs (Copaxone, Betsaseron, Tecfidera). Diabetes taught him discipline, but discipline did not control MS. Every new brain scan (MRI) showed new inflammation (enhancement). The medications were not working.

Before HSCT, Patrick was using a cane to walk short distances and a wheelchair for longer distances. He kept falling, could not read, and had blurred vision, bilateral hearing loss, urine retention (neurogenic bladder), paraplegia (weakness of one arm and leg), and chronic pain. Before MS, he was working in a hospital and was a nursing school student. MS made it impossible to do either. He sold his car because he could not use its manual transmission. Everything in his life was being stripped from him.

Patrick had been dealt a double whammy: two chronic diseases—childhood-onset type 1 diabetes and adult multiple sclerosis. I was uncertain how much of his neurologic disability was diabetic neuropathy versus MS. I cautioned him that HSCT would not help diabetic neuropathy and that he may not improve. In truth, I did not want Patrick to have unrealistic hope. I wanted him to be skeptical of a possible benefit from HSCT. Because of the risks involved, I would always intentionally undersell HSCT. He chose to go ahead with it, and now seven years have gone by since his transplant.

After the transplant, everything improved. Patrick regained all function and now walks without assistance; in fact, his gait became normal. He can even run. Bilateral ear ringing (tinnitus) resolved. His vision corrected with readers (reading glasses). His balance normalized, allowing him to walk on his tiptoes for the first time in a decade. He is planning to return to nursing school and, based on his own life experience, become a specialist in pediatric endocrinology (diabetes).

When Patrick was enrolled for HSCT, Illinois Medicaid had approved his treatment. I knew the medical director, and Illinois Medicaid had always approved HSCT. Medicaid paid below cost so the hospital lost money on each Medicaid transplant but helping the patient in front of me—not the money—was what was important. After we had already collected Patrick's hematopoietic stem cells and scheduled his HSCT admission, Medicaid sent me a letter reversing its approval for transplant. I could not believe it. I called Patrick, called the hospital, and called the director of Medicaid, who informed me that Patrick's Medicaid had been switched to the Affordable Care Act (ACA) coverage. I told him that Patrick had already been approved and that the transplant was in progress. He said there was nothing he could do, but a few days later the director called back and told me that Patrick could proceed with HSCT. He also told me that this would be the last approval and that never again would Medicaid give approval for HSCT.

After that, several of my patients called me and told me that their Medicaid had been switched to ACA coverage without their consent or input. I called the medical director to find out what was going on. I was informed that there was no one available to speak with me. Since then, Medicaid has always denied HSCT.

In case you were wondering, HSCT did not affect Patrick's insulin requirements. There is not enough space in this book to go into detail, but HSCT can reverse adult-onset type 1 diabetes if transplant is performed early after onset (within six weeks). (For more information, go to www.astemcelljourney.com.)

Lost to Follow-up

A patient once came to me from another state. He was self-employed and had switched his private medical insurance to the most expensive premier ACA plan. He told me that he did this because ACA promised the best medical coverage at the best price. I told him I did not think so, but we would try. We submitted for HSCT approval. They denied it. There was no appeal process or person to speak with. His transplant never happened. He moved overseas and was lost to follow-up.

Anonymous Medical Director

The medical director of an insurance company gave me permission to use his name, but because I want to protect confidentiality, I'll call him "Anonymous." Anonymous has been a medical director of a major medical insurance company from the time I started prescribing HSCT treatments for autoimmune diseases more than twenty-five years ago. Throughout the decades, I intermittently spoke with him on behalf of individual patients. More often than not, he was able to provide the company's approval for transplant. Even when that was not possible due to policy changes, it helped to convey a patient's situation and the most recent publications and state of the art in the field. To change minds, you first must have someone to speak with who is willing to listen.

Being able to speak to a person who accepts responsibility and has authority is the first and most important key to solving any problem. Even if the answer remains *no*, it plants a seed that may germinate at some future date. One to two years after publication of my randomized MS trial, this medical director sent me an email saying, "I should reach out and tell you that, at long last and due to your work and some pushes from some others, I will be approving autologous stem cell transplant benefits for selected members with MS."

Anonymous cautioned that insurance approval may remain iffy and variable. He also said that insurance companies and most physicians lump all transplants together in their minds. They do not understand that the toxicity and outcome depend upon the treatment (conditioning) regimen and the patient selection. Anonymous was preaching to the choir.

Many good people, including some people in the insurance industry, have contributed to this field. They have done so without expecting their names or contributions to ever be recognized. The key to approval is being able to speak with a person who accepts responsibility and accountability for the policy and the decision for denial, and to make them see my patient as a person instead of a number.

One Last Word on Secondary Progressive MS

As I've mentioned, HSCT will not benefit patients with late secondary progressive MS (SPMS). As a caveat, SPMS with enhancing MRI lesions that indicate ongoing active inflammatory disease is called active SPMS (aSPMS) and may still demonstrate some partial reversal of neurologic disability after HSCT. SPMS without recent enhancing MRI lesions, called nonactive SPMS (nSPMS), does not reverse neurologic disability after HSCT. It is my current belief that patients with nonactive progressive MS will need a different stem cell with neuro-regenerative potential instead of HSCT-induced immune regenerative effects. I'm working on it.

Wingman

Keith worked as a United States Geological Survey research engineer. In his free time, he owned and managed a cattle ranch and was an avid scuba diver and fisherman.

Due to numb fingers, minor left foot drop, and balance issues, he was diagnosed with multiple sclerosis and was started on self-injecting MS drugs, with no benefit. Keith did his own research and found information about stem cells on the Internet. At one of his next neurology appointments, he brought up the subject of stem cells. His neurologist said that he thought stem cells would probably be the answer to MS, but that we "weren't there yet." The neurologist was partially right. We were not there yet for SPMS. But we were there with HSCT for RRMS.

Keith's wingman from his college going-out-for-drinks days had become a hospital president later in life. When Keith turned to his friend for advice, his friend said that he supported the concept of HSCT. Keith had entered early progressive MS, for which immune-based therapies (HSCT is a type of immune therapy) would be much less effective. His transplant was uncomplicated. While everyone's experience varies, Keith said going through HSCT was like having a mild flu. Improvement was, however, more gradual than with most patients, but after several months, Keith returned to part-time work and started a physical therapy routine while continuing to work on his ranch.

Over the next five years, Keith's MRI images showed no new lesions, but only minor neurologic improvements occurred. On every return visit, Keith would bring me and my staff fresh ocean fish that he speared while scuba diving off the Caribbean and Florida coasts.

Keith was the first person to introduce me to lionfish, hogfish, and triggerfish, all of which taste surprisingly good.

Keith is now nine years post-transplant. He retired from work but still runs his cattle ranch, helps on his parents' farm, and continues to fish and scuba dive. The numbness in his fingers did resolve and the MRI shows no new lesions, but due to the progression of foot drop, he started using a cane. Keith feels that without transplant, he would have been in a wheelchair by now. I listen to my patients. I learn from them. In the future, it might be reasonable to design a lower intensity regimen without risk of fever (as fever may further exacerbate nerve injury) for early SPMS with enhancement on the MRI, that is, aSPMS.

Keith is a lighthouse beacon, helping other patients and inspiring me to keep going. He correctly argues for HSCT sooner rather than later and encourages me and other patients to "never, never, give up."

Is HSCT Totally Safe?

Is HSCT totally safe? The answer is *NO*. Each patient must be warned of this, in writing and verbally. Risks are disease- and regimen-specific, but for RRMS, significant risks associated with a nonmyeloablative regimen are infections, infertility that is age-dependent, and ITP (low platelets that clot blood) occurring within the first two to three years after HSCT. There is also the concern that a patient, in hopes of getting HSCT, will not mention other disease-related conditions they have that may increase transplant complications. In the early days of HSCT for MS when myeloablative regimens were used and patients were selected with SPMS, the mortality (as reported by the EBMT) was greater than 5 percent. With appropriate patient selection (RRMS and no other coexisting major illness) and a nonmyeloablative conditioning regimen, the risk is now approximately 0.2 percent.[21] In the most recent report of over 500 patients undergoing HSCT, mortality occurred from comorbid disease (coexistent sickle cell disease) and failed hospital infrastructure/

support (legionella bacteria growing in the hospital water supply).[22] The hematopoietic stem cells have no role in efficacy or toxicity. There are currently several myeloablative and nonmyeloablative conditioning regimens being used for HSCT of MS (Table 4).

Conditioning regimen	Stem cells purify before reinfusion	Myelo-ablative	Toxicity	Cost
busulfan, cyclophos-phamide, antithymocyte globulin	Yes	Yes	++++	++++
BEAM (carmustine, etoposide, cytarabine, melphalan), antithymocyte globulin	Yes	Yes	+++	++++
cyclophos-phamide, antithymocyte globulin	No	No	++	++
cyclophos-phamide, rituximab	No	No	++	+

Table 4. Qualitative schematic differences between hematopoietic stem cell transplant (HSCT) trials for releasing-remitting multiple sclerosis

The most aggressive conditioning regimen is an intense leukemia regimen (busulfan, Cytoxan, and ATG) that is used in Canada. A less intense but still aggressive myeloablative regimen is BEAM and ATG originally developed for lymphomas that is currently used by several American centers. Two nonmyeloablative, less intense, safer, and less expensive immune targeting regimens that the majority of people have been treated with worldwide are cyclophosphamide and ATG or cyclophosphamide and rituximab.

Presented herein were the stories of patients undergoing immune specific nonmyeloablative regimens, which should beg the question: why take the risk with a more intense and toxic myeloablative regimen? I've written this book to make sure physicians and patients know that they have options.

While not without risks and while relapse may occur, HSCT is the first and only treatment to convert relapsing remitting multiple sclerosis (RRMS) into a reversible illness in which most patients remain drug free for the long-term with remissions now exceeding one to two decades. With proper patient selection and optimal nonmyeloablative regimen, this one-time treatment has changed the natural history of RRMS. Unlike drugs, it has improved neurologic disability and improved quality of life and is cost-effective compared to continuing drugs.

Dr. McFarland, the retired Chief of Neuroimmunology at the NIH, had cautioned me before I began this marathon that everyone who had tried to cure MS had failed. Following HSCT using a non-myeloablative regimen for RRMS, most patients have not relapsed. As demonstrated in these patient stories, many patients are now ten to twenty-one years post-HSCT, with remarkable return of neurologic function, no further treatment necessary, and no evidence of MS activity since HSCT. I still refrain from using the word *cure* and depending on conditioning regimen about 23 percent of patients relapse, but perhaps we have finally found the right door for patients with aggressive RRMS to enter. Notably, this was undertaken as an academic altruistic pursuit with no anticipated financial reward or licensed patent.

Medical publications are, by necessity, detached, dry, and loaded with data and statistical analysis; they do not contain the human story. If physicians, administrators, and insurers could have gotten to know these patients and lived their human stories, the stone-cold skeptical cynicism and resistance to this approach would have been short-lived and would have evaporated a long time ago.

CHAPTER 5

SYSTEMIC SCLEROSIS: TURNING INTO STONE

I was in my first year fresh out of medical school when I first encountered a patient with systemic sclerosis. In those days, being an intern meant working all day, every day, for six to seven days a week with in-house night call generally every third night, except when working in the medical intensive care unit (MICU) or emergency room (ER), when night call was every other night. Thirty-six sleep-deprived, hectic hours in the hospital, twelve hours at home, then back to the hospital to start all over again. I was in the first year (internship) of my medical residency. The surgical residents had it worse. Surgical intensive care unit (SICU) was one month of every day and every night call. During that month, a surgery resident could not go home, leave the hospital, or even leave the unit. They had to arrange for a spouse, relative, or friend to pay their bills and take care of their home. Food and fresh scrubs were brought to them in the unit.

Baylor College of Medicine and its SICU were under the control of Michael DeBakey, MD, a world-renowned heart surgeon. The residents, whether medical or surgical, just called him Good Old DeBakey (GOD). Today this sounds like some sort of United Nations OCHA (Office for the Coordination of Humanitarian Affairs) workplace violation, but he pushed himself harder than he pushed us. We respected him, and thought of ourselves as professionals, not employees, so we voluntarily emulated him and followed his example.

The surgical residents started their first year as kind, likable individuals, but by the end of that year, they were basically jerks. Nevertheless, I understood and did not hold it against them. Medical residents accomplished the extraordinary. Surgery residents did the superhuman. The environment changes you because failure to adapt is career suicide. Pure determination, drive, and focus take over. Pleasantries and small talk evaporate long before the end of the first year. Today this sounds inhumane, and such long training-work hours are now a thing of the past. On the flip side, this prolonged Parris Island Marine Corps Boot Camp training makes you an excellent doctor and develops within your subconscious an instinct and a sense for disease that no textbook can match.

The half-joke we told one another during residency training was that if you go home at night to sleep, you will be missing half the cases. Paraphrasing Virchow, the father of human pathology, "To study a disease without books is to sail an uncharted sea, while to study books without patients is not to go to sea at all." As a patient, you may not want a doctor who is chronically sleep-deprived, but when your life is at risk and you need help, you are grateful for a doctor who has the instincts, skills, and knowledge honed from being trained under those conditions.

It is unbelievable what the body can accept as normal if the mind is determined to push through. I learned firsthand that you can adapt to and function for decades in stressful situations with chronic sleep deprivation. More importantly, I learned what the body and mind can do from my own patients, who fought incurable disease with courage and a resolve to keep fighting despite, short of a miracle, having zero chance of escape.

Green Eyes

It was about 2:00 a.m. when the nurse paged me to see a patient who was "short of breath." When I arrived at the bedside, in front of me was a seventeen-year-old girl with thin, long, straight brown hair, green eyes, and tanned skin. But the tanned skin was not a suntan. She was afflicted with a disease called systemic sclerosis (also known as scleroderma). Her skin was rock-hard with no flexibility and while most areas were brown, there were patches of albino (depigmented) skin color. She was on nasal cannula oxygen, which is saying that pure oxygen was being provided by a plastic tube that had been inserted into her nose. Her breathing was difficult and labored due to scleroderma involving her lungs, but her eyes sparkled with determination to live. Her mother and father were each on either side of her bed, hovering over her. They were afraid and frustrated and would have, without hesitation, traded places with her, but there was no one in the room who could barter such a trade.

In truth, I did not know what to do. Except for giving her more supportive care (more oxygen), none of us knew. I called the second-year resident and woke the attending doctor, who was at home. When you do not know, do not be too proud or too embarrassed to get help. There was, however, nothing available but supportive care. No help existed. We were all impotent.

Because the patient's fingers were contracted, I held her hand as best I could and talked to her softly, reassuring her in a calm voice. Although I have never read a scientific study on this, there is value in a calm, reassuring voice and in human touch, especially when someone is in distress. As the reclusive chess master Bobby Fischer said on his deathbed: "Nothing eases suffering like human touch." She was perceptive and knew that my words were a bluff. Despite frozen hands, she closed her fingers the few millimeters that they could still move around my hand and looked at me, too out of breath to speak sentences. Her eyes reflected gratitude, as if to thank me for trying to hold on to her in this world. We got her, or more accurately she got herself, through the night. I went off to another service that morning.

Two weeks later, she was dead. She never was allowed to experience the anticipation of a prom dance, a marriage, or a mother's love for her own children. Her parents had endured the worst fears of their lives, to helplessly watch their child die. Millions of years of evolution had instructed their genes to fight to the death for their child. The night I met them, they were tense, like a cornered animal would be, ready and wanting to fight, to do something, anything, in a last stand to free their daughter. I felt useless; it was like watching a family dart back and forth looking for an escape from their raft just before it slipped over Niagara Falls.

An invisible knife passed through me when I learned that she had died. Decades later as I look back, I cannot remember her name, but my memory pictures her in front of me as if it had just happened last night. What happened to her was not right. It was not fair. But when you take care of people who get disease through no fault of their own, you quickly learn that life is neither evenhanded nor fair. It is a gift that can be revoked at any time and needs to be appreciated while we still transiently hold it.

Whether by chance or by fate, or if you are so inclined to believe in life after death by her intervention, later in life a light went off in my mind about a new type of treatment that may stop and reverse systemic sclerosis. When this light went off, it ignited a fire in my gut to see it through. This is the story of hematopoietic stem cell transplantation (HSCT) for systemic sclerosis, a disease (like other autoimmune diseases) in which your own immune cells attack your own body.

Turning into Stone

Ninety percent of patients with systemic sclerosis—a chronic and progressive hardening of the body's soft tissues—are young or middle-aged women. When the skin is diffusely involved or when the lungs are involved, the percentage of disease-related death is high. It causes the destruction, distortion, and loss of small blood vessels and capillaries. Patients often use the colloquial name *scleroderma* (pronounced skleh-ruh-DUR-muh), which means "hard skin," but other rare diseases also cause hard skin so in medical parlance it is referred to as systemic sclerosis. Out of deference to my patients, I will use the terms *scleroderma* and *systemic sclerosis* interchangeably.

With this disease, the skin becomes leather-hard without elasticity. You cannot pinch it. The joints progressively contract, slowly tightening, drawn in and permanently flexing in a closed position (Figures 1A and 1B). It is like watching an ice skater spin faster and faster as they draw their arms and legs in, except they cannot reextend their arms outward to stop the tailspin their life has entered.

Scleroderma not only hardens the skin, it also hardens the vital internal organs with progressive and potentially lethal involvement of the lungs, kidneys, gastrointestinal tract (gut), and heart. For reasons nobody knows, the skin of a patient's back remains normal and unaffected in systemic sclerosis.

Despite the seriousness of their disease—which transforms them into a frozen, stonelike, contracted statue with shortness of breath, progressive slow suffocation, a failing heart, severe reflux into the esophagus causing constant heartburn, gut stasis and malabsorption, skin ulcers that may extend into the bone, and kidneys that may fail

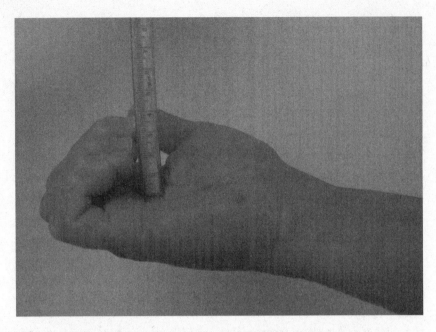

Figure 1A. Example of a scleroderma hand that cannot completely close. The ruler quantitates how far the fingers can close as the gap between fingers and palm.

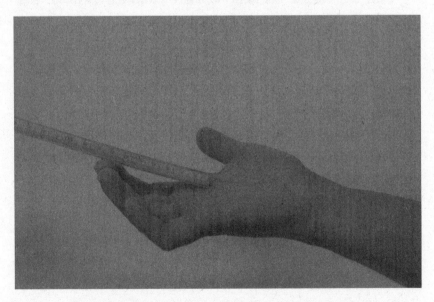

Figure 1B. Example of a scleroderma hand that cannot open completely. The ruler quantitates the distance that the fingers can straighten.

at any time—patients with scleroderma rarely complain. Despite being trapped in a medieval horror film with their life being stripped away from them, scleroderma patients have always impressed me as being notably stoic and resilient.

Their pulse is frequently irregular. Yet they almost never mention feeling palpitations (abnormal heartbeats) unless you specifically ask. They may only be able to walk a few feet at a time because of shortness of breath, or they may be in a wheelchair with a nasal cannula oxygen compressor strapped under it. Yet they generally do not complain about their shortness of breath. In a casual, nonchalant, passing remark, one patient graphically described scleroderma as the feeling of a "baby anaconda snake inside my body growing stronger and contracting around me a little tighter each day."

Cleverness and dry British humor have been attributed to a British cultural emphasis on public civility, self-control, and maintaining "a stiff upper lip." Scleroderma patients literally have the proverbial stiff upper lip. Their entire face loses elasticity and becomes stiff to the point where their mouth cannot open enough to bite a sandwich or eat a cheeseburger. The nuanced range of emotions most of us can convey through facial gestures, twitches, and winks is lost. Scleroderma patients live the lexicon of "chin up" and "soldier on" in the face of a relentless and worsening hardship. Nonverbal facial expressions of anger, surprise, love, fear, sadness, and joy are gradually replaced by an expressionless mask. Yet behind the mask of scleroderma, a patient's eyes can still sparkle with a passion for life, showing that they are not willing to accept their fate. Systemic sclerosis patients are the only people I know who are happy to see wrinkles and creases return on their skin. As I learned after starting HSCT for patients with scleroderma, improvement usually starts quickly after the procedure. Before leaving the hospital, most patients can usually pinch and lift their skin for the first time in years.

Designing an HSCT Trial for Systemic Sclerosis

Systemic sclerosis with diffuse skin involvement or when involving the lungs has a mortality rate of around 5 percent each year. The typical patient is a young woman. When I first started HSCT for scleroderma in the late 1990s and early 2000s, there was no effective therapy for the disease. The only drug that was reported to benefit systemic sclerosis was cyclophosphamide (also known as Cytoxan). The *New England Journal of Medicine* (*NEJM*), the highest-ranked medical journal in the world, published an article that Cytoxan was effective for scleroderma lung disease.[1]

NEJM reported the results of the Scleroderma Lung Study, which was a randomized trial of oral Cytoxan, a commonly used immune suppressive drug, taken daily for one year compared to a daily placebo (basically a sugar pill) also taken for one year. The duration of taking Cytoxan was limited to one year because when taken long-term, Cytoxan may cause bladder cancer and the blood cancers myelodysplasia or leukemia. To document lung function, the study followed the forced vital capacity, which is a measure of how rapidly the body can move air out of the lungs. After one year, the forced vital capacity worsened compared to enrollment baseline by 1.0 percent when taking daily Cytoxan and worsened by 2.6 percent when taking the placebo. The study concluded that one year of daily Cytoxan had a beneficial effect for scleroderma lung disease.

The problem with the conclusion of beneficial effect for lung disease is that the lungs did not improve. The lungs in reality got worse; they just not did decline as fast as compared to people who were getting nothing (placebo)—a 1 percent decline versus a 2.6 percent worsening, respectively. Another problem with the interpretation that the lung "benefited" was that the DLCO, which measures the ability to move oxygen between the lungs and blood, decreased (worsened) more (minus 4.2 percent) in the Cytoxan group than in the placebo group (minus 3.5 percent). The greater decline of DLCO after a year of Cytoxan was minimized because it did not reach a statistically sig-nificant difference between the two arms (Cytoxan versus placebo).

The two-year follow-up of this *NEJM* study was reported one year later in 2007 by the same group in a less prestigious and thus less-read journal, the *American Journal of Respiratory and Critical Care Medicine*.[2] The two-year follow-up reported absolutely no difference in the worsening of lung function (and skin tightness) between Cytoxan and placebo. There was no significant or numerical difference in the decline in lung function (FVC or DLCO) between daily Cytoxan compared to doing nothing.

After two years, patients receiving Cytoxan worsened at exactly the same rate as those taking a placebo, yet because of this *NEJM* publication, many scleroderma patients worldwide were subsequently treated with daily oral Cytoxan for scleroderma lung disease.

A young, bright rheumatology fellow who had come from Rome, Italy, to study with me regurgitated one morning on rounds that oral Cytoxan improved lung function in scleroderma. So we decided to discuss those articles in journal club (a meeting to critically review recent articles in the academic literature). During journal club, I witnessed the light go on in her eyes. I have always loved seeing a young mind absorb new material and connect the dots. I also saw the sense of disbelief that she felt at being misled by the original *NEJM* publication.

Patients are never enrolled all at once in a trial. As stated in the 2006 *NEJM* paper, patients had been enrolled between 2000 and 2004. At the time of the 2006 *NEJM* publication reporting the one-year follow-up, many patients already had two-year data. By doing two papers—the one-year data showing a slowing of decline in lung function and the two-year follow-up paper showing no difference in rate of lung deterioration compared to doing nothing—all the data was honestly presented, but the way it was presented had misled people.

Due to the workload, the amount of material to learn, and the pressure to care for patients, young doctors often have little free time to read an entire article. They jump to the summary paragraph at the end of an article or, worse, turn to Google to source information and knowledge. The further information is removed from the research and the actual data, and the more voices filter the data, the more misinformation arises.

Per the second law of thermodynamics, the law of entropy, disorder always increases the further you are from the source (original data and research). For that reason, I always tell students to do the opposite—that is, first read the methods and results section of a manuscript. The second secret to becoming a good doctor is that you should always look under the microscope at pathology specimens and at any imaging studies, whether X-rays or CT scans or MRIs, along with the pathologist or radiologist. You will learn more about your enemy (disease) if you go to the source and look it in the eye. Do not let someone else tell you what the enemy looks like. Look at it yourself!

I was once helping an internationally known European pulmonologist (lung doctor), who is an expert on the scleroderma lung, write a book chapter and noticed that he regurgitated the same reiteration of the conclusion from the 2006 *NEJM* article that daily oral Cytoxan improves lung function. I pointed out that the lung function did not improve; it declined (just not as fast as doing nothing). I also pointed out that the two-year data by the same group showed no difference compared to doing nothing, as both worsened equally. I sensed the light go on in his brain as well. He was impressed and suggested that we write a review together. I appreciated the suggestion, but I knew it would not happen because we both had too many other pressing obligations. I have found that correcting professionals engenders two types of reactions. One is gratitude for taking the time to question group-accepted concepts (groupthink). The other is the human equivalent to the response of a threatened animal: the baring of sharp canine teeth, the extending of claws, and the bristling of hair on the back of the neck. The fight game is then on.

My Italian rheumatology fellow, upon returning home to Italy to complete her training, had to take a written and an oral examination to pass her fellowship. When her professors corrected her by stating that oral Cytoxan improves scleroderma lung function, she quoted the actual results from both articles. Her teachers had to look up the original articles. She passed the exams, as the idiom goes, with flying colors. I am so proud of her. I hope she knows that.

For scleroderma, I knew that daily oral Cytoxan, as given in the *NEJM* article, was, in general, not very effective. Higher doses of intravenous monthly Cytoxan were also standard of care for scleroderma and appeared to be more effective than daily oral dosing. Because Cytoxan was and still is considered a standard of care for scleroderma, I designed the transplant conditioning regimen to include much higher doses of Cytoxan given daily over four days. Whether a drug is effective or not depends on the details of how it is used, including the dose administered and how it is given.

Since the 1960s, transplant doses of Cytoxan have been regularly used for hematopoietic (blood) stem cell transplantation of the autoimmune disease called aplastic anemia. Cytoxan is cheap, patent-expired, and safely dosed daily for four consecutive days to a total dose of 200 mg/kg (50 milligrams per kilogram body weight per day), so that was the dose I chose for transplant of systemic sclerosis. I also used an anti-immune cell protein (antibody) called antithymocyte globulin (ATG) that was also used for transplant of aplastic anemia. This regimen is, as were most of the regimens that I designed, a non-myeloablative regimen. (For a video on the HSCT procedure, go to https://astemcelljourney.com/reflect/purpose/.)

Bulletproof

One of my early scleroderma patients was referred to me by the rheumatology service from another American university. Tucker was the classic man's man, friendly and charismatic but tough as steel. He owned his own construction firm. When once confronted by someone with a gun, he exhibited nerves of steel and refused to back down. I myself agree with police recommendations to give up your money, but on that day, Tucker took a chance and fortunately luck favored him. Mary, his wife, told me, "Tucker is the strongest person I ever met. He is bulletproof."

Tucker's self-confidence to take on the world was turned upside down at age fifty-eight by scleroderma, a disease that attacked from inside his bulletproof vest. While 90 percent of scleroderma patients are women, 10 percent are men, and the disease can be quite severe for many men (as well as for women). One day he awoke with stiffness that never went away. This progressed to rock-hard skin covering his body, constricting his movements, and confining him to a wheelchair in a contracted shell of a body. His rapidly progressing disease did not respond to traditional doses of Cytoxan, and after being evaluated at a well-known medical university, he returned home with the advice to get his will in order, as he probably would not live for more than a year.

Tucker prayed that he would die quickly to end the unrelenting pain and relieve the psychological havoc that had been forced upon his family, who were helplessly watching him suffer. Scleroderma is an invisible assassin that enters unexpectedly, unannounced, and unseen into your life. I have often been amazed by the psychological resilience of women, and Mary, Tucker's wife, was no exception. She did not back down from this assassin and was determined to fight to her last breath. She searched the Internet and found an article in *Reader's Digest* about a patient of mine with scleroderma who had experienced remarkable improvement after HSCT. She tracked down the patient featured in the story, who referred her to me. Mary informed her local physician what she had discovered and asked him his thoughts on HSCT. He was unfamiliar with the concept, but given the dire circumstances, told her to go ahead and try it.

For Tucker, HSCT was difficult, and increased oxygen was required to get him through. But the day after stem cell infusion, the stiffness was already improving and his hands were opening up. Within a year he was back running his company and riding a motorcycle. A decade after transplant, he remains normal without medications. He said, "Every day before the transplant, life was being slowly squeezed out of me, while every day after transplantation is like an injection of life back into my arm." Once on a telephone follow-up, one of his originally skeptical rheumatologists who saw him post-HSCT said in astonishment, "This sh*t really works."

Commodore

Keith was a naval officer and commander of a destroyer. I always referred to him as "Captain." Regardless of military rank, when at sea, the commander of a war ship is the captain and when at war or if the ship is in peril, the captain's authority is absolute and unquestioned. He is responsible for that ship and the men and women under his (or her) command. Above all, Keith was a gentleman.

Once he told me that the worst feeling in his life was when he was asked to speak at the funeral of a sailor who had committed suicide. After that memorial service, the last meeting of every day, no matter how late or how busy he was, no matter what hotspot in the world his destroyer was deployed in, Keith always met with the ship's medic to ask if anyone was depressed or had suffered loss or separation of a spouse or family member, or was feeling alienated or isolated, or otherwise was having troubles. Keith owned his job. He owned his destroyer. He would have been a great doctor if he had chosen that career.

A lot goes into commanding a destroyer. It is a mobile independent unit that is highly electronic. It sees, tracks, and can annihilate an enemy beyond the horizon. It needs to defend the fleet, and it needs to function independently on its own. Any captain, in order to be comfortable when isolated alone at sea, needs to know how the ship works both inside and out.

Keith was tall, muscular, and ran marathons. One day he could not finish a race. He attributed this to a bad day. The next time he tried to run, he could not. He had to stop because he could not breathe, and his hands were tightening up. He was diagnosed with scleroderma and relieved of his military command.

I have always found that the military takes good care of active-duty personnel, and Keith was no exception to this commitment to medical excellence for nonretired service men and women. The Navy medical facilities (Walter Reed/Navy Bethesda) had no experience with HSCT for scleroderma, so Keith was referred to me. He had skin that was tightening, but his main problem was shortness of breath. His lung function tests were steadily declining, and the imaging studies (chest X-ray and CT scan) showed worsening lung disease.

After the transplant, everything started to reverse for Keith. He began to run again and was placed back on active duty, although it was limited to desk duty. Then one day after HSCT, he got an order from the Chief of Naval Command: "Report to your immediate superior at Pearl Harbor Naval Station for duty as the commanding officer of the destroyer USS . . ." He had won his battle against scleroderma. He had gotten his life back. Keith invited me to be present for the change of command ceremony. It is a rare honor and every part of me wanted to attend, but I had sick patients undergoing HSCT in the hospital. I was the only physician in my division, and I had my own duty to my patients.

Keith has continued with his naval career, healthy, on no medications. I regret not being there for the change of command and doubted that I would ever have that opportunity, that honor, again. Most recently, Keith was promoted to commodore, a naval rank for command of more than one ship. A squadron of eight naval destroyers is now under his command. Ten years after HSCT, he mailed me his commodore command pin and cap with a thank-you note. Such an honor is normally bestowed only on a sailor or soldier who has saved your life in combat.

Imprisoned

Darlene, a thirty-six-year-old optimistic, positive-energy woman, was diagnosed with scleroderma a few months after the birth of her second child. The cause of scleroderma is unknown and whether its onset was related to delivery of her second child or was a coincidence is unknown. One scleroderma researcher once documented male lymphocytes (immune cells) in the blood of women who had given birth to male babies. But it was never proven that those male immune cells caused the scleroderma, and women who have never been pregnant also develop systemic sclerosis, as do men.

Scleroderma overwhelmed Darlene with a feeling of physical and spiritual ugliness. She lost her independence and lost her friends. Worse yet, she lost herself. She felt as if no one could love her. It became impossible for her to care for her children or to be a loving wife to her husband. Darlene forgot what it felt like to be beautiful and to have patience, self-esteem, and confidence. Scleroderma not only destroyed her physically, it crushed her psychologically.

When Darlene arrived in clinic, she was in a wheelchair with contracted fingers, hands, and arms. Her legs were contracted at 90-degree right angles and could not be straightened. She could not stand even with assistance. Her skin was rock-hard, and scleroderma had destroyed her kidneys. Due to her rock-hard skin, a vein could not be cannulated for vascular access to perform intravascular hemodialysis. Since venous access was not possible, she was on peritoneal dialysis with a tube sticking out of her board-hard abdomen. The peritoneum is the smooth lining or sac under the belly's skin and muscles that surrounds the organs within the gut.

Darlene's husband had to pick her up out of her wheelchair and carry her to the exam table, where she sat with her contracted legs off the table as if she were still in the wheelchair. When I pushed her chest back to a reclining position, her legs would go up into the air, frozen with a 90-degree bend in her knees. She was a surfboard on a teeter-totter. Push either end down, and the other end went up. Her fixed hand and arm contractures meant that Darlene could not feed herself or wipe herself after toileting. Whichever family member was present had to do it for her. Ulcers had eaten through parts of her body, including her buttock (perisacral) region, elbows, knees, and heels.

The disease destroyed who Darlene was and how she felt about herself. She had turned into stone. Amazingly, it had not yet completely conquered her spirit. Her eyes still betrayed her determination to live. A human soul still hung on, locked inside the prison of a frozen body from which no medicine offered the hope of a pardon.

Because scleroderma causes the lungs, kidneys, and heart to fail, I was accustomed to scleroderma being a complicated and difficult transplant. But I had never taken on such an end-stage case. There had to be limits to what HSCT could do. I had not yet had enough experience, and I was not sure that an autologous HSCT would work. Despite the severity of her skin and kidney disease, Darlene's lungs and heart checked out OK (well, marginally OK). Darlene had a healthy sister who was an immunologic match (termed an HLA match) and who became her stem cell donor.

The transplant was difficult, and Darlene was slow to recover. With the conditioning regimen I used, most people recover their blood counts (the process of which is called *engrafting*) on day nine after infusion of hematopoietic stem cells; she did not engraft until day sixteen, and afterward she was transferred to a rehabilitation facility. She still needed her usual twenty-four-hour care for feeding, toileting, and turning in bed (she could not roll to her side). She did not manifest the instantaneous predischarge improvement that occurs with most patients. I regularly saw Darlene in rehab and was beginning to think that the transplant had failed. But slowly her skin started to loosen. Scleroderma often begins distally on the fingers or toes and progressively over time ascends up the arms and legs to the face, chest, and abdomen. After HSCT, improvement may first be appreciated where it first started (e.g., on the hand), but scleroderma may also retreat from the area most recently involved, with improvement descending down the limbs, as was the case with Darlene. It took time, but by the end of a year she could walk without assistance, although initially she was hunched over.

To get off dialysis, her sister, who had donated the stem cells, donated one kidney. A chimera is a Greek mythological creature composed of two creatures, and in medicine we use the term *chimera* for a person who through transplantation is partly another person. Because Darlene was already an immune chimera from HSCT and already shared her sister's immune system, she did not need and did not receive immune suppression or other drugs to prevent rejection of her sister's kidney. Her sister's kidney has functioned in Darlene normally for more than a decade without any ongoing immune suppression. Darlene no longer needs dialysis. Her skin has continued to loosen, and she no longer requires any assistance. She started driving a car and sent me a video of her carrying her own groceries to and from her car. For over a decade, she has remained free both of scleroderma and dialysis and is on no therapy at all.

Darlene has returned to feeling like a beautiful woman and a wife, with two children who are now young adults.

Why We Needed a Randomized Trial

I witnessed these responses over and over in my patients after HSCT, but the medical community would not accept the results. I was not a rheumatologist (nor a neurologist), much less accepted within the field of rheumatology as a scleroderma subspecialist. Like all cliques, it is a small, tough group to be invited into. In truth, I did lack their training pedigree. Talented, dedicated, and hardworking rheumatologists have spent their entire careers researching and studying this disease. It seemed unlikely that a non-rheumatologist dropping in from out of the clear blue sky could accomplish such a feat. It is normal human nature to view such a coup d'état with skepticism, especially when it comes from a nontraditional direction.

HSCT also struck several in the rheumatology community, which by tradition is focused on bench research and outpatient care, as too intense and too dangerous for an inpatient procedure. The patients, however, did not perceive it that way. Patients did not want to be imprisoned in their bodies nor endure the constant threat of further bodily injury and death from the stealthy and unrelenting assassin called scleroderma. I empathize with the patients' perspective.

The resistance of the medical community is understandable because they were not doing what I was doing. In the movie *Avatar*, the expression "I see you" was used to convey that you understand. Since HSCT was developed outside of the traditional subspecialists, they literally did not "see it." We were in different worlds, and when something seems too good to be true, it is appropriate to be critical. Mary, Tucker's wife, mentioned to me years later that if she had not seen with her own eyes how much her husband had improved, she would not have believed it was possible.

Some implied that this was done for media attention, financial motives and incentives, or that we were offering false hope. Nothing could be further from the truth. These studies were done with no financial reimbursement or any future copyright privilege or possibility of a license or financial gain.

The media, nonphysician organizations, and others not directly working with stem cells at the patient bedside had spent a decade hyping stem cells without clinical results. For those of us doing the work, or at least for me, I was reticent to talk with the press and never advertised or sought media interviews. In fact, it was the opposite—the media sought me out when we published in the more prestigious medical journals because the journals had press releases accompany an important publication.

Early on in this process, I decided not to participate in the lay media frenzy. As a consequence, a "journalist" from a respected newspaper informed the university public relations office that if I did not speak with him, he would trash me in the article and never publish anything good about the university again. I was naïve and did not realize that this could happen or that someone could be so righteously malevolent. The university did not seem surprised. They offered to stand by my decision, but they strongly advised me to speak with the journalist. I had no intention of negatively impacting my patients or the university. I did the interview.

The patients' testimonies and my talks and publications, along with the lay media reports, helped with public awareness, but generally within the established professional world, my words fell upon skeptical ears. Patients would ask me, "Why isn't the administration standing on the rooftops shouting this out and supporting you?" I never answered, as I remained perplexed by this too. I was viewed by some in the hospital as a free radical, but the university provided me academic independence, and that was all that I needed.

On one occasion a transplant surgeon said to me, "People in the hospital do not get you. They think you are either crazy or a genius." What they did not get is what motivates me. What motivates me is not a big office or salary or title. It is my patients. They came from all fifty US states, as well as from around the world. As a solo physician, I worked around the clock, available to patients 24/7. Watching them get better from this treatment was my motivation. My reward was seeing the idea I had conceived become a reality. The big salary, title, and office did not compare to seeing people who had been failing at other major medical centers get back the health they thought had been lost forever. For me, it was not a nine-to-five job. It was a passion. While the administrators sat in big offices with fancy new furniture, I had to scavenge for the money to pay for my office space, which had no windows and mismatched used furniture that had been discarded by others. But for me it was OK. What I was doing was more important.

I also learned from my patients that our medical system far too often fails them. And I learned from individuals with titles after their name that success may cause outward projection of a jealous antipathy from those who are so inclined. Professor William Burns, my Johns Hopkins mentor from when I was a fellow, once told me, "Focus on your original research and publications. That is what is important." So I did.

I am a trained university academician. I knew that falsely believing that a therapy works may arise from unintentional expectation bias by the patient and by the investigators, especially if the measured outcome parameters are subjective. For scleroderma, my outcome parameters—e.g., survival, lung function tests, and imaging performed by staff without knowledge of treatment—were less likely to display expectation bias. But without a randomized trial, patient selection could still bias results.

Because my scleroderma transplant patients did not improve or worsened on standard medical care options, then manifested remarkable post-HSCT improvements, a selection bias seemed unlikely. Still, the best way to avoid selection and outcome bias is randomization and, if feasible, blinding, so neither the patient nor the physician knows which treatment is being given. In order to make HSCT for systemic sclerosis accepted within both the subspecialty and broader medical community, I had to do a randomized trial. There was no choice but to do it the right scientific way.

Conducting the Randomized Trial

Since this type of improvement and reversal of disease after HSCT had never previously been reported with any prior treatment for scleroderma, for the randomized trial, I continued using the same transplant conditioning regimen of Cytoxan and anti-thymocyte globulin (ATG). I named the trial ASSIST, an acronym for American Scleroderma Stem cell versus Immune Suppression Trial. Patients with scleroderma who had a shortened life expectancy (that is, those with significant skin tightness and/or lung disease) were randomized to either hematopoietic stem cell transplantation or to the best standard of care accepted by the rheumatology community—i.e., monthly intravenous Cytoxan. Designing such a trial is tricky. To ethically perform a randomized trial, the two treatments must have equipoise—that is, the efficacy of the two therapies should be roughly equal.

It is unethical, or should be unethical, to give one group of patients highly effective therapy and another group ineffective therapy, especially for a lethal disease such as systemic sclerosis. On the other hand, if we did not perform a randomized trial, a skeptical academic community would never acknowledge HSCT as a viable treatment. I got around the problem of equipoise by allowing patients who were randomized to monthly intravenous Cytoxan but failed to improve to have the option to cross over to HSCT.

The results of ASSIST were published in *The Lancet*, one of the most prestigious peer-reviewed medical science journals in the world, and were also presented at several professional medical conferences. It was the first randomized control trial of HSCT for systemic sclerosis or, for that matter, any autoimmune disease.

Scleroderma patients on the control arm of ASSIST received the standard therapy (intravenous Cytoxan), but their skin and lung function still worsened, just as they did in the *NEJM* study using oral Cytoxan. In contrast, for patients randomized to HSCT, their skin and lung function significantly improved above baseline enrollment. For the first time in medical history, a randomized trial for scleroderma showed real improvement, that is, reversal of disease with improvement in organ function in the patients receiving HSCT, not just slowing the disease progression (i.e., slowing the disease worsening).

After HSCT, the patients remained off immune-based therapies. Patients who had been on the control arm of monthly Cytoxan when switched to HSCT had the same reversal of disease and improvement in their skin and lung function. It was not only more ethical to allow a crossover for those failing the control arm, but the patients on the control arm (Cytoxan) became their own controls, failing on monthly Cytoxan but improving after HSCT. Compared to pretransplant baselines, quality of life (in medical parlance, SF-36) markedly improved after HSCT but not on standard therapy (intravenous Cytoxan).

Nurse and Patient

When she received her transplant, Sharon was in her thirties with two young children. Prior to the onset of scleroderma, she had been living a successful and normal life. She and her husband, Craig, are both from the Midlands in the UK, where they met in nursing school, first becoming lifelong friends, then getting married, and together completing their training in nursing. They left the Midlands in the 1990s to start their nursing careers in America and became American citizens. Craig specialized in medical intensive care and Sharon in gastroenterology.

Sharon and Craig both speak with a characteristic Brummie accent. Both had always worked at the same hospital. What Sharon wanted from life was to be a good nurse, a good mother, a good wife, and someday a good grandmother. Scleroderma threatened to upend all of that. She had the familiar scleroderma symptoms of swollen hands, tight skin, fatigue, cough, stiffness, contractures, Raynaud's (parts of the body such as fingers turning white, blue, and purple from loss of blood flow), and dyspnea or shortness of breath.

As medical professionals, Sharon and Craig read the published standard of care (Cytoxan) data and were not impressed. When evaluated for the randomized ASSIST trial, they argued against Sharon being randomized to standard therapy with Cytoxan. Craig was especially determined to get his wife what he viewed as the best therapy. I explained how we had to do a randomized trial with the outcome data collected by someone other than me or this therapy would never be accepted. I explained how promising treatments, when put in a randomized trial, may surprisingly fail to show superiority. I gave them a come-to-Jesus talk explaining how potentially dangerous HSCT could be compared to monthly Cytoxan.

It is important to inform patients verbally and in written consents (Institutional Review Board-approved) about the risks of HSCT, the most serious of which is death. Because the conditioning regimen drops blood cells (red blood cells, platelets, and immune cells such as neutrophils and lymphocytes) to virtually zero, life-threatening anemia (lack of oxygen), bleeding (lack of blood clotting), or infections (lack of immune cells) may occur. Anemia can be prevented by red blood cell transfusions. Bleeding can be minimized with platelet transfusions. Infections can be minimized with antibiotics. But there remains a small but real risk of these getting out of control. Infertility or inability to have a baby after HSCT may occur, depending on regimen and patient age. The risks depend on the conditioning regimen and are more severe with myeloablative regimens compared to nonmyeloablative regimens. The disease itself may also increase organ-specific risks. Specifically, scleroderma patients, due to disease-related damage, as will be discussed later, are at risks of heart failure, kidney failure, or gastrointestinal (gut) bleeding.

These arguments about toxicity did not hold water with Sharon and Craig. They were well-educated medical professionals who well knew the risks of HSCT. So why did they insist on HSCT? It is because scleroderma has a mortality of 5 percent per year (when high skin score or lungs are involved) and, in general, organ damage is only slowed (not reversed or stopped) by drugs. They felt like they were being sold the London Bridge and were not buying it. Inside, I agreed with them. If it were my wife or daughter, I would demand to get the transplant also. I was losing the argument, but I had to do the randomized trial. If you meet eligibility for a trial, you must be randomized. You cannot be treated off-study on a compassionate basis because doing so would introduce bias (conscious selection) and nobody would accept the results. I would not.

In the clinic that day was a chair of the Institutional Review Board (IRB) that regulates and monitors protocol conduct. I flagged him down and asked for his help. He read Sharon and Craig the riot act and made clear that it would be a randomized trial or the highway. They accepted the randomization and, as fate would have it, Sharon was randomized to the monthly control arm of Cytoxan. They were disappointed. The saving grace for Sharon and for the study was that if your disease progressed—that is, if you were failing (worsening) after one year of standard of care (intravenous Cytoxan)—you would be allowed to get HSCT. Nevertheless, continued scleroderma-related organ damage could make the transplant more difficult and make it harder for the transplant to salvage these failing organs or to facilitate a return to normal function.

Sharon got worse on Cytoxan. After one year, she was allowed to receive HSCT. Craig stayed in her room throughout the transplant. Medically, he was a blessing for me as well. Besides the usual regular nursing-floor care, Craig was a twenty-four-hour MICU nurse at Sharon's bedside. The transplant was not easy, and they missed the birthday of their eleven-year-old son. After transplant, Sharon's skin improved, her lungs improved, her shortness of breath disappeared, and she returned to being a nurse and caring for patients.

After HSCT, Sharon and Craig arranged for me to speak about this technology at their hospital. After my talk, they introduced me to their sons. Before going to medical school, I had double majored in chemistry and mathematics, and I remember how interested in mathematics and how bright and inquisitive their sons were. For the older son who had already had some math classes, we talked about different aspects of math for thirty minutes. More than a decade later, Sharon and Craig still work as nurses, their eleven-year-old is now a naval aviator fighter pilot, and their youngest son is in college.

About a year after Sharon's transplant, Sharon and Craig took me on a nature hike. As we hiked, they gradually got farther and farther ahead of me. I could not keep up because I was the one getting short of breath on the uphill incline. Sharon, who before the transplant had experienced shortness of breath from scleroderma lung disease, was breathing comfortably and hiked well ahead with ease. Watching them leaving me behind, I was proud of the results of HSCT.

In a switch of roles, they were worried about me. I brushed it off and told them not to worry. Inside I knew that I was sacrificing my health for my work. As the Dalai Lama said, "The young sacrifice their health for money. The old sacrifice their money for their health." I was on a university salary, so my sacrifice was not for money; it was to make the idea of HSCT for autoimmune diseases a reality.

In 2013, I was invited to present my ASSIST randomized trial on HSCT for scleroderma data, which had been published in *The Lancet*, at a meeting on stem cells at the Vatican in Rome.[3] Many distinguished university professors, business leaders, some members of the European parliament, and a Nobel laureate were speakers at the meeting. I was allowed to select a few patients to tell their stories, one of whom was Sharon. It had taken me years to become comfortable speaking in public, and I was worried about my patients having stage fright. However, they were naturals, completely at home on the stage.

At the Vatican meeting, there was no religious indoctrination or trying to convince anyone of anything. (A couple of speakers even spoke about their research with embryonic stem cells. I, too, have worked with embryonic stem cells in my lab.) I have presented in many academic meetings, including ones at Harvard and Cambridge, and this was one of the best academic meetings that intergraded multiple viewpoints and disciplines. I was able to bring my then-high-school-aged son, and I witnessed the light and passion for science go on in his eyes during this meeting.

A bioethicist from an American university had also been invited to speak. His first words were a joke about a pedophiliac priest in the Catholic Church. It was like starting a teachers' convention with a joke about teachers being convicted pedophiles. It seemed so inappropriate in so many ways. The cardinals in the audience remained polite and quiet.

After the meeting, the bioethicist speaker got into an exchange with Sharon and Craig. When they pushed him how he could ignore the data and their personal experiences with scleroderma and HSCT, the bioethicist responded that he did not agree with the risks involving adult stem cells. What this bioethicist missed was not only does an individual have a right through informed consent to decide their own treatment, but that I was the one who had been arguing for decades against the National Institute of Allergy and Infectious Diseases's (NIAID's) more aggressive and toxic myeloablative conditioning regimens for autoimmune diseases.

For more than twelve years, Sharon has remained free of any further skin or lung recurrence of scleroderma. The only residual intermittent problem that many patients retain, though often with less severity, is Raynaud's syndrome, which in Sharon's case caused a slow-to-heal leg ulcer about eleven years after HSCT.

Gathering More Data: ASSIST II

Because the interim analysis on the ASSIST randomized trial was so significantly and statistically in favor of HSCT, we stopped enrollment on the randomized ASSIST trial, published results, and continued doing HSCT for scleroderma on a larger number of patients, all of whom went directly to HSCT. Those results were published two years later again in *The Lancet*.[4] The data on improvement of skin, lungs, and quality of life held up in the larger cohort of patients and over a longer interval of time.

Teamwork

Cyndy contacted me from California. Her problems began when she noticed difficulty running a marathon or scuba diving with friends. She could not catch her breath, and her muscles would ache and spasm. Tight skin, heartburn, bloating, diarrhea, rectal bleeding, vomiting, and loss of weight ensued. At first, the hard skin removed Cyndy's wrinkles and made her look younger. But the early youthful appearance of hard, smooth skin was a Faustian trade to which she had never agreed. Tight skin limited movement, including breathing, dressing, bending over, chopping vegetables, opening mail, and opening her mouth wide enough to eat a sandwich. All became progressively more difficult. Picking something up off the floor became impossible. Scleroderma patients have told me that when they accidentally drop money, they just leave it on the ground because it is too difficult and painful to pick up. If they get down on the floor, they may be unable to get back up.

Shortness of breath was no longer something that happened only when Cyndy was trying to run or scuba dive. It happened when she was walking from the car to her front door. Long daily naps replaced talking with friends. Brain fog made it impossible for her to continue working. Words got mixed up in her head. Her medical team of five doctors prescribed a plethora of drugs for her different symptoms, but all the drugs seemed to have little or no impact. Cyndy was trapped inside her body with an incurable disease. She often cried and thought a lot about what would happen to her daughters, grand-children, and husband.

This was the turning point. She and her husband, Bill, had a habit of tackling problems through teamwork—taking on projects, working hard, and solving problems together as a team. They wanted to stop this disease and had heard about HSCT from a friend in their support group who had undergone HSCT for scleroderma. So was the state of the field early on. Most often, patients learned of HSCT from other patients, friends, or the lay press, not from their local physicians or healthcare providers. They learned about the two clinical trials underway at the time—our nonmyeloablative protocol and a myeloablative National Institute of Allergy and Infectious Diseases (NIAID) protocol using total body irradiation.

What many physicians did not realize and needs to be reemphasized is that not all transplants are the same. The early and late toxicity (and efficacy) is due to the conditioning regimen (and patient selection). The autologous (your own) stem cells are simply a supportive blood transfusion. Once understood, I always found that patients who were aware of the alternatives did not want to be part of the NIAID trial.

Patients did not want to be exposed to total body irradiation in the conditioning regimen of NIAID's trial because of long-term late side effects, including leukemias and cancers. Conversely, patients randomized to the Cytoxan arm did not want to be forever excluded from receiving HSCT in the NIAID trial. If randomized to the control arm of Cytoxan, the NIAID trial (called SCOT for Scleroderma Cytoxan Or Transplant) excluded patients from receiving HSCT, even if the Cytoxan failed. Why did NIAID exclude patients from ever getting HSCT if they continued to fail on standard Cytoxan? The reason is that NIAID could not compare the primary study end point of death between the two arms if a crossover to HSCT was allowed in patients randomized to the standard Cytoxan group. I know, as I was there and argued to allow crossover to HSCT during the development of that trial.

In the end, most informed patients came to the same conclusion, preferring a nonmyeloablative, nonradiation-based regimen with a crossover to HSCT if standard therapy continued to fail. Two patients with life-threatening disease progression in the Cytoxan control arm of NIAID's SCOT trial subsequently came to me because their test centers were contractually forbidden by NIAID from performing a transplant.

Cyndy's transplant was difficult, and her worsening shortness of breath during the transplant was a problem. She needed supplemental oxygen. It was a slow comeback, but after HSCT everything improved, with most symptoms improving within the first year. And like most patients, further less dramatic improvements have continued to evolve over subsequent years. Her skin softened, her movements returned to normal, and her mouth was able to open normally again. Her Raynaud's and heartburn did not go away completely, but they did fade into the background noise of a normal, everyday life.

At day one hundred post-transplant, Cyndy ran in a 5K race. When breaking through the finish line tape, she shouted, "I'm back!" Two years later, she hiked the Grand Canyon with her husband and a group of ten friends. Since HSCT, she has hiked the Sierra Nevada and Madre Mountains and the Swiss Alps. She only notices shortness of breath when she hikes above 10,000 feet.

The Scleroderma Foundation was an integral part of Cyndy's recovery. It was there that Cyndy and Bill learned everything they could about scleroderma, including learning about specialists and HSCT clinical trials. Cyndy became a member of the local chapter's board of directors, and Bill joined the Scleroderma National Foundation board. They wanted to share their knowledge to help other patients. In 2011, the Scleroderma Foundation arranged a session in which the two competing HSCT clinical trials—one with my nonmyeloablative conditioning regimen (ASSIST) versus one with NIAID's total body irradiation myeloablative conditioning regimen (SCOT)—were allowed to debate the pros and cons of each conditioning regimen. I was very grateful for the opportunity as the society's meetings had been heavily influenced by the NIAID SCOT myeloablative trial and discussion of nonmyeloablative ASSIST had hitherto been taboo. Cyndy and Bill helped to remove that taboo and opened the eyes of a lot of good people in the National Scleroderma Foundation.

After HSCT in 2012, Cyndy started a Facebook group called Scleroderma Stem Cell Pioneers for patients that is focused strictly on HSCT for scleroderma. Today the group has over three thousand members, averaging thirty-three new members per month, and hundreds of HSCT patients use the group to share their experiences with other patients to help them understand what HSCT is and is not, if they may be a candidate, how to find a center, and in general feel supported throughout the arduous process. Because of Cyndy and Bill's teamwork to start the Scleroderma Stem Cell Pioneers Facebook group, talk at conferences, post YouTube videos, and serve as board members in the Scleroderma Foundation, thousands of scleroderma patients from around the world have learned about nonmyeloablative HSCT.

It has been more than a decade since Cyndy's transplant. Bill and Cyndy are now semiretired. They are living their lives as the team they were always meant to be. They hike and scuba dive together. They invest their time and energy into their children and grandchildren, but they still also help scleroderma patients.

Collegiate Athlete

Before scleroderma, Aeron was a six-foot, six-inch tall, 210-pound college athlete. Being graceful on the court or on the field came easily to him. He was diagnosed with scleroderma during his last year of college. It became impossible for him to move quickly or smoothly, to have energy, or to even compete in sports. The magic was gone, and with its departure, plans for a professional athletic career vanished. Scleroderma turned his life around 180 degrees.

After the onset of scleroderma, Aeron tried to work with either juvenile or adult offenders or people with special needs. He loved people, and if he could not play sports, he wanted to help others who needed help. But scleroderma was not finished with him. Soon any type of work became impossible, and Aeron had become the person who needed help. His weight dropped from 210 to 120 pounds. He could not look up or down, look to the left or to the right, or sit up. His fingers and elbows were contracted. He had bilateral shoulder subluxation (partial dislocations). His upper arms had slipped partially out of the shoulder sockets. It looked painful, but like other scleroderma patients, Aeron never complained. His knees were bent at 90-degree angles, his back was hunched over, and his neck was flexed with his face planted looking permanently down. Whether in a wheelchair or on a scooter, he could not look up. By rotating his eyes up into his skull, he could see a few feet in front of his scooter. No matter how hard you pulled on one of his limbs, none would relax or straighten. It was like trying to straighten bent steel.

Aeron's hands and elbows were contracted. He could not use a spoon to put food in his mouth and could barely open his mouth to take a full bite or even to smile. His face was drawn and unrecognizable to people who had known him before scleroderma. He no longer had friends with whom he socialized. His companion became a black Labrador retriever named Lilly who always stayed by his side. His smooth pre-scleroderma skin was splattered with white patches and was rock-hard. Bandages covered ulcers on his fingers and elbows. Due to severe gastric reflux into his esophagus (GERD), he could not lie flat on a bed. He slept in an upright recliner.

The hardest insult to his dignity was having to rely on help for everything—cleaning, cooking, showering, toileting, shopping, dressing, eating. His own skin was strangling him. It kept relentlessly tightening.

During the first week after his stem cell transplant, Aeron's skin immediately started to loosen and while still in the hospital on Thanksgiving morning, he was able to flex his wrist normally. It was a Thanksgiving Day to be thankful. Over the next few years of rehabilitation, he was able to perform yoga, Pilates (named after the German Joseph Pilates), boxing, Lameco Eskrima (a Filipino martial art), water aerobics, and recumbent bicycle riding. Although his mobility is not completely normal, his mouth, legs, and back improved, and he is able to stand up straight.

Aeron participates in adaptive downhill skiing. He passed his driver's test and is able to drive again. Recently he has returned to work full time and has dedicated his life to advocating for others with disabilities.

In 2019, he was invited to Washington, DC. The National Scleroderma Foundation had arranged for him to meet with five senators to advocate for more money to be given to NIAID. The irony not told is that I had walked away from the NIAID monies and their approach using myeloablative total body irradiation and accomplished Aeron's results with no funding and using a different, less expensive and less toxic conditioning regimen without the risk of radiation-induced leukemia and cancers and had published the results (in *The Lancet* 2011 and 2013) almost a decade before NIAID published (in *NEJM* 2018). Money is a solution, but money is also the problem.

Aeron showed the senators his before and after slides. The senators could not believe it. While the slides were powerful, Aeron wished that he had videos of himself before HSCT. He did not because he had never thought that improvement would be possible. Years later,

Aeron can still see gradual improvements and is socializing with friends again. His canine companion during the dark years of scleroderma, Lilly, remains faithfully at his side.

Rosy the Riveter

When Rosy was a teenager, her doctor told her that she would never be able to have children. After being told that, she buried herself in blue-collar work, like a real-life Rosie the Riveter. Rosy was a hard-working, fair-minded, honest, good-spirited, salt-of-the-earth woman who worked in factories and in coal mines.

Between the ages of thirty and forty, she developed hearing problems and started wearing hearing aids. Her hearing loss was attributed to sucker and blower fans in the underground coal mines that were so loud that she could barely hear herself think.

She went on to get her state mining papers for Mine Examiner, Mine Manager, Electrical Hoisting Engineer, and her EMT-D license. Later she worked at a strip mine, which is an above-ground coal mine. The giant, 190-ton coal trucks that she drove were as deafening as jet engines.

Rosy worked in the strip mine of a small town until age fifty-three, when she got whiplash from one of the rock trucks. A year later she was diagnosed with black lung from decades of inhaling coal dust. At age sixty-one, she developed scleroderma. It progressed rapidly with her main symptoms being fatigue and hard skin over her hands, arms, legs, abdomen, and chest. She could no longer bend over and had difficulty opening her hands. It took forever for her to get dressed. She could only walk one block before needing to stop and rest from weakness and shortness of breath.

Rosy had always done jobs traditionally done by men and was independent and self-sufficient. She told me that she would do anything to avoid scleroderma forcing her into a nursing home.

Her transplant took place in 2011 at the age of sixty-three. Her lung scan showed both coal miner's lung and scleroderma lung. Given the coexistent black lung from coal, I did not know if I could help her, and I told her so. She wanted to go forward with the transplant anyway, as she really had no other medical options and could not continue as she was. She did fine throughout the transplant.

By six months after HSCT, Rosy's skin hardness had decreased 50 percent from a pre-HSCT modified Rodnan skin score (mRSS) of 42 down to 24. Within one year, the skin in her arms had returned to normal. She could walk one mile on a level treadmill and could bend over. The chest pain from esophageal reflux (heartburn) went away, and her Raynaud's markedly improved.

About three years after HSCT, she developed a low-grade follicular lymphoma that has remained in remission for the last six years. At age seventy-three, more than ten years post-transplant, Rosy continues to live alone in her own home, cuts her own grass with a riding lawn mower, drives to the grocery store, and cooks and cares for herself. Recently, when I spoke with her, I was touched and surprised that her concern was for me and for how I was doing, not for herself.

Medic

Katrina was a combat medical technician (medic) for the British Army. She was deployed with the British Armed Forces in Iraq and had married her lifelong friend, who was also in the British army. Upon returning home, she left the army (with honor) and began working as a civilian in a hospital surgical suite in the United Kingdom.

In 2008, Katrina was diagnosed with scleroderma and came to America to undergo HSCT in 2014. At the time of HSCT, she could no longer work and had given up her job. She was too stiff to stand up without assistance. Her doctors advised her to get a wheelchair, but she refused. Her walking was limited due to severe aching, soreness, and pain in her legs. When deployed into an active combat arena, you worry about being taken prisoner. Katrina never thought that scleroderma would be the commandant that imprisoned her inside her own body. She was trapped by tight, nonflexible skin and limited upper and lower limb joint mobility. Scleroderma-related gut issues ranged from digestive dysfunction that alternated between constipation and diarrhea to postprandial (after eating) stomach bloating that limited the amount and types of food she could tolerate.

The UK National Health Service had not recognized HSCT as a treatment for scleroderma and would not pay for it to be done there or in America. As a veteran, Katrina reached out to the British Army, but they also declined to pay. She was trapped not just by her disease but also by the government-run medical system. She reached out to the public for funds. Local newspapers and television ran with her story. People from all over England came to her support. Money even came in from Australia and from a few people in America.

After HSCT, Katrina's fatigue and digestive issues disappeared. She was able to eat a normal diet. Her skin loosened, her mobility improved, and her walking became normal. It is now seven years since HSCT, and she has returned to working part time. Her hobbies include snowboarding, bicycling, and stand-up paddleboarding. Her husband remains a member of the British military.

In 2014, Katrina was told by British physicians and the National Health Service (NHS) bureaucracy that HSCT did not work, and that it was not an option. By having her story in numerous newspapers such as the *Daily Mail* and *The Telegraph*, Katrina's effort helped change the professional opinion toward HSCT within the UK.

While the British Broadcasting Corporation (BBC) declined to carry her story, Independent Television (ITV) was all over it. In the UK, ITV is as big as the BBC. Katrina recently said to me, "Today the conversation has changed; British doctors are now open to the idea, and patients are more informed of their options." During that conversation, eight years after her HSCT in America, I was struck that Katrina's concern and wishes were for me, not for herself.

In fairness to the British medical system, one UK hospital had tried HSCT for scleroderma, but it was a disaster and the hospital stopped doing it after two early cardiac (heart) deaths. Because so many people, including physicians, do not seem to understand the concept behind HSCT for autoimmune diseases, it is important to reemphasize that the common thread of the procedure and for which it is named—"stem cells"—is a misnomer. Stem cells have no therapeutic role. The hematopoietic (blood) stem cells are nothing more than a blood transfusion, a supportive blood product to ensure or hasten recovery from low blood counts. The efficacy and toxicity depend almost entirely on two things: the conditioning regimen and patient selection. In those early days, the importance of scleroderma involvement of the heart was underappreciated by virtually everyone (including myself). The British hospital scleroderma deaths arose from a conditioning regimen that was too heart-intense as well as the wrong patients being selected for that heart-intense regimen.

The Potential Risks of HSCT for Scleroderma

I and my colleagues at the University of São Paulo (Brazil) reported in *The Lancet* 2013 the outcome on more transplants for scleroderma than any other study even to this day.[5] While the same post-HSCT long-term improvements with disease reversal and drug-free improvements in skin flexibility, joint movement, lung function, and quality of life occurred, five of ninety patients died. They were heart-related (cardiac) deaths. The families of these patients, in an unexpected reversal of roles and gracious manner, comforted *me* for trying to help their loved one. They knew that their loved one would rather die trying to reverse scleroderma than to continue suffering a slow death from total body strangulation. Still, I felt responsible for each death. I knew that I could not do HSCT for scleroderma if I could not predict who had such bad hearts that they could not survive the treatment. Despite all that was accomplished, I once again felt impotent, just as I had that night during my residency when I was called to evaluate the seventeen-year-old scleroderma patient with shortness of breath. After all this time and success, I felt that I was right back where I had started—not knowing what to do—in this case, not knowing how to identify high-risk cardiac involvement before HSCT.

It's a Matter of the Heart

In 1992, President Bill Clinton's campaign strategist, James Carville, ran a successful presidential election on the slogan: "It's the economy, stupid." Well, when it comes to scleroderma: "It is the heart." By sitting at each patient's bedside 24/7 (I was the only physician in my small division of one physician), I figured out that a cardiac catheterization with fluid challenge helped exclude some patients with significantly impaired hearts. Basically, there are three big problems that the scleroderma hearts suffer from: 1) pushing against high pressure in the lungs; 2) a stiff heart that has trouble relaxing; and 3) inflammation with or without fluid around the heart and/or constriction of the sac around the heart.

Scleroderma inflames and slowly destroys the lungs, causing the pressure required to pump blood into the lungs to rise, a phenomenon that in medical jargon is called *pulmonary artery hypertension* (PAH). The right side (chamber) of the heart pumps blood through the lung and into the left side (chamber) of the heart. The left chamber of the heart pumps blood to the body. High lung pressures from stiff pulmonary arteries cause the right side of the heart to fail.

If lung pressure is too high, the heart is at high risk of failing during HSCT. Some people use ultrasound (an acoustic probe held on the chest) to determine pulmonary pressures, but for scleroderma, ultrasound is too often not accurate. A cardiac catheterization is required for accuracy. To get an accurate pressure reading, a catheter is inserted through the femoral vein in the groin into the right heart and then the pulmonary artery. The problem is, without a fluid challenge, even a cardiac catheter reading can be falsely reassuring. Patients remain with no oral food or liquid intake (NPO, or nothing per mouth) since midnight before the heart catheterization, which is often not performed until later in the afternoon. Their pressures may be falsely reassuring because they are intravascularly dry by the time of the procedure. When one liter of normal saline is infused over ten minutes, a normal person's heart pressure readings do not change, but the heart pressures of a person with scleroderma may rapidly rise. Like their skin, their blood vessels are stiff and nonelastic. If the heart pressures are too high, they will not tolerate a transplant.

Scleroderma is an immune-mediated disease of the blood vessels. Small blood vessels spontaneously spasm shut, causing the blood flow to stop. This results in a phenomenon called Raynaud's syndrome, which is named after the French physician Auguste Gabriel Maurice Raynaud, who first described it in 1862 in his doctoral thesis. Small vessel constriction causes tissue areas such as the fingers to first blanch white from vasospasm due to no blood flow (Figure 2) followed later by a purple color from lack of oxygen and then red from reactive opening of the vessels (vasodilation) and return of blood flow.

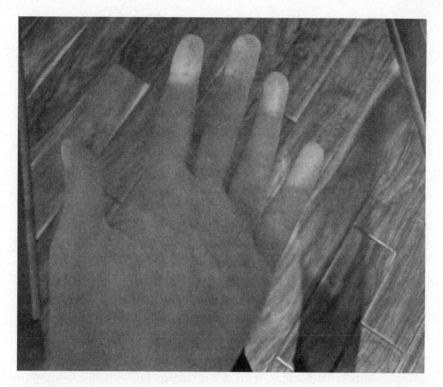

Figure 2. Raynaud's syndrome is common in systemic sclerosis but is not unique to systemic sclerosis and may occur with or without other diseases or symptoms. Small vessel constriction causes the digits (fingers) to first blanch white (vasospasm with no blood flow), followed later by purple (lack of oxygen from vasospasm), and then red (reactive vasodilation).

In scleroderma, Raynaud's syndrome also attacks the heart, which is the largest vascular (blood vessel) organ. The result is small areas of fibrosis (microfibrosis) within the heart muscle and a stiff heart incapable of relaxing (called diastolic dysfunction). The stiff heart is just like the stiff skin and joints. Both joints and heart can contract but cannot relax normally.

I also discovered that cardiac catheterization cannot always pick up this heart stiffness. I had always looked at all pre-HSCT cardiac magnetic resonance imaging (MRI) studies with a radiologist, but none of us knew what to look for at the time. I remember the cardiac

MRI of a patient who did poorly and whose heart had an odd septal motion that the radiologist did not think was pathologic. The two chambers of the heart are connected by one common wall called the *septum*. I restudied the MRIs on all patients and realized that septal flattening during relaxation (diastole) or, even worse, a septal bounce, indicated a stressed heart that would not tolerate HSCT. I taught the reading room radiologists how to look for this, but because they changed every few weeks—often to a new fellow in training—I had to teach each new radiology fellow and ask that the finding be included in the report. Fortunately, I always reviewed every cardiac MRI in person with the radiologist.

Professor Dominique Farge is a seasoned, talented French physician who is one of the original pioneers in HSCT for scleroderma and other autoimmune diseases and who was the coprincipal investigator in the European randomized HSCT trial for scleroderma. An outside monitoring committee ascribed deaths on that trial to fluid in the lungs (pulmonary edema) or to many organs failing (multiple organ failure).[6] I called Dominique as those were symptoms of heart failure, which was the factual cause of death. Dominique immediately understood what I was saying. She wrote up and included me on new European guidelines for pre-transplant scleroderma heart evaluation that included doing a cardiac catheterization with fluid challenge and MRI imaging of the heart.

The failure to aggressively work up the heart before transplant occurred in early days of HSCT because heart failure was not recognized as the leading cause of death by scleroderma experts. Every time I listened to a rheumatology (muscle and joint) doctor or pulmonology (lung) physician, they all said that the leading cause of death was lung injury. These are organ-specific (joints or lung) specialists and extremely bright but with focused visual fields. That is the problem with being a member of a highly specialized, small group of experts. "Expert" thinking gets into group thinking. As Abraham Maslow, a psychologist known for his theory on self-actualization, said, "I suppose it is tempting, if the only tool you have is a hammer, to treat everything as if it were a nail."

It is true that the lung is a major cause of morbidity, and scleroderma patients may end up on oxygen due to bad lungs. But scleroderma patients do not, in general, die from lung failure. That is, they do not die from suffocation. The ultimate cause of death is heart failure. And during a transplant with high-dose Cytoxan, the main cause of death is heart failure. I knew this because I sat at every patient's bedside. HSCT is such powerful therapy that it exposes the pathophysiology of a disease. To emphasize this point, I wrote an editorial about scleroderma titled, "Scleroderma: it is a matter of the heart."[7]

Water Kills

In the first *Jumanji* movie, the character played by Robin Williams says, "A lot of water kills." For scleroderma patients, a little salt water infused in the vein can kill (Figure 3).

Scleroderma patients often have impaired hearts, a fast heart rate, and low blood pressure, which in a normal person would be indications for intravenous salt water (normal saline), but those are not necessarily indications for patients with scleroderma. Fluid going into a stiff scleroderma heart may back up in the lungs, causing more shortness of breath. In general, treatment should be a water-removal pill (diuretic) to decrease blood volume. This low blood pressure may be misunderstood in a hospital setting, resulting in not just fluids but also the use of a potent vasopressor drug such as Neo-Synephrine to artificially increase blood pressure by further constricting blood vessels. In scleroderma, the small blood vessels are already abnormally twisted and pathologically constricted, which is why the fingers of scleroderma patients turn white, purple, and red (from Raynaud's syndrome).

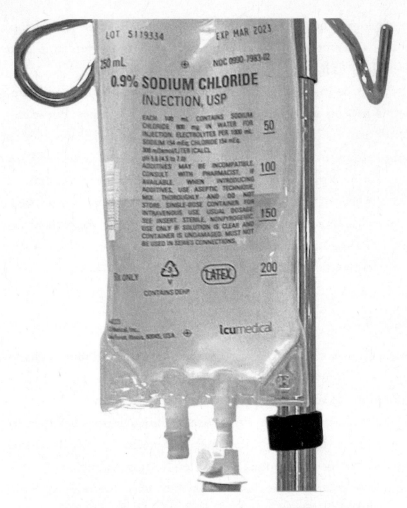

Figure 3. What is viewed as a completely harmless and innocuous bag of normal saline (salt water) when aggressively infused into the veins of a patient with systemic sclerosis may precipitate heart and lung failure.

A patient of mine with scleroderma walked into the hospital but later that night died after having been started on both IV fluids and Neo-Synephrine (a potent vasoconstrictor) to elevate her blood pressure. The autopsy showed a massive acute circumferential heart attack that extended all the way around the heart and from the bottom to the top of the heart. The coronary arteries were normal. There was no atherosclerosis, and there were no plaques or obstruction in her coronary arteries.

Since my patient's coronary arteries were normal, why did she have a massive heart attack? Scleroderma hearts are prone to vaso-spasm and vasoconstriction (Raynaud's of the heart). Scleroderma, combined with fluids and a vasopressor such as Neo-Synephrine, may cause the entire heart to infarct. Neo-Synephrine is such a potent vasoconstrictor that it carries a black box warning not to be given by bolus injection, which is how that patient was treated—by bolus fluids and bolus Neo-Synephrine.

One college-aged scleroderma patient called her brother because she felt like she was getting the flu. Her brother took her to the emer-gency room of the hospital of the university where she attended classes. As is a general standard practice, the ER physicians started a normal saline infusion in her vein. As the patient became short of breath and progressively more unstable, the doctors gave her more fluids and then ordered her brother out of the room. She was a young, idealistic col-lege girl who had walked into the emergency room with her brother without assistance or shortness of breath. Within hours after starting fluids, she died in the emergency room alone and separated from her brother by the hospital staff.

The medical community has failed to recognize or emphasize that the scleroderma heart is stiff and cannot tolerate sudden fluid infu-sions or shifts. Physicians see a scleroderma patient's stiff skin, but what they do not realize is that their stiff skin equals a stiff heart. Because of problems like this, I kept my pager on and next to me and took calls twenty-four hours a day, seven days a week, for twenty years, and in so doing almost lost myself.

I also put on the wall of every scleroderma patient's room a sign reading, "No intravenous fluids. No vasopressors." I also told my patients not to allow intravenous salt water or new medications with-out insisting that I should be paged, even it was two in the morning.

CAST: A Heart-Safe Protocol

Despite the success of the Cytoxan/ATG regimen in treating sclero-derma, scleroderma hearts with certain pretransplant features could not tolerate a high-dose Cytoxan regimen. I declined to transplant patients with pretransplant high-risk cardiac findings, much to those patients' disappointment and protestations. Even some scleroderma patients who met the heart criteria still had a tough course.

Cytoxan at the doses we utilized for scleroderma has been used for transplant of the autoimmune disease called aplastic anemia from the 1960s until the present day. Aplastic anemia patients have normal hearts. Similarly, multiple sclerosis patients have normal hearts and tol-erate Cytoxan without experiencing heart problems. In scleroderma, the heart, even when the workup reveals normal function, is virtually always impaired to some extent. I did pre-HSCT cardiac catheteriza-tions with fluid challenges, echocardiograms, and magnetic imaging of the heart, but current technology is not sensitive enough to predict an uncomplicated safe transplant with absolute 100 percent certainty. Needing to establish a safer regimen for scleroderma patients, I wrote a new protocol for patients who had significantly impaired hearts.

The new regimen decreased the Cytoxan dose from 200 mg/kg to 60 mg/kg and added another immune-specific drug called fluda-rabine that has been in use for at least forty years to kill immune (lymphoid) cells. The anti-immune cell protein anti-thymocyte glob-ulin (ATG) stayed at the same dose while two doses of Rituxan, an anti-immune B cell-directed protein, was added. The new regimen was called CAST, an abbreviation for CArdiac (heart) Safe Transplant.[8]

This had become a three-plus-decade process of refining and improving the regimen for scleroderma (and other autoimmune dis-eases). But every time I started a new regimen and new protocol, I spent at least one to two years of work in designing, writing, and getting approval before enrolling a patient. As a fellow at Johns Hop-kins, the Fred Hutchinson Cancer Center, and the NIH, I was taught to design my own protocol, and that remained my approach through-out my career.

It came as a surprise to me that over time, progressively more and more physicians treated patients without a protocol or used a protocol designed by someone else, usually a Big Pharma company, that was managed by an outside office. This trend accelerated over my career to the point where most people had no idea what I was doing designing my own protocols and standard of care pathways. Hospitals depend in part upon physicians generating money for them. Creating a pro-tocol, although it was the right thing to do, was time-consuming and not a directly measurable revenue-generating activity.

I know that if you cut corners, more mistakes happen. Writ-ing your own protocol forces you to do your homework before you start, to study the disease, research the literature, seek input from specialists, circumvent and develop contingencies for complications, design enrollment and exclusion criteria, create a treatment pathway for nurses and pharmacists to follow, and establish outcome crite-ria to monitor. A good sailor, no matter how experienced, does not just jump into a boat and sail away. They will study the navigational charts, study the weather, plot the course, and become familiar with electronic and manual navigation before setting off. Even despite all my preparation, whenever I started a new protocol, there was always the worry of the unknown and unforeseen going wrong. Unlike sail-ing, where you wait for good weather, in HSCT you sail directly into the storm with very sick patients. In addition, every patient is differ-ent, and there are often multiple variables at play.

To learn about a disease and a patient, you have go to the source and look at the test results you ordered. I always did as I was trained. I reviewed every scleroderma chest tomography (CT) imaging scan and every heart magnetic resonance image (MRI) with a radiolo-gist. The radiologists were always welcoming to me. We learned from one another. They did not know my patients' clinical histories, and my input sharpened or changed their reports. For me, each meeting with a radiologist was an opportunity for free one-on-one teaching. Radiologists often sit in dark booths in dark rooms, looking at computer screens for hours at a time. I think some of them appreciated having human company when I would drop in to review a case.

Initially, I only enrolled patients on the CAST (cardiac safe transplant) protocol who were excluded for heart reasons from receiving the ASSIST regimen (Cytoxan 200 mg/kg/ATG). The CAST regimen (Cytoxan 60 mg/kg/fludarabine/ATG/Rituxan) was, even by scleroderma standards, surprisingly nontoxic. Patients with scleroderma-impaired hearts tolerated treatment surprisingly well. The main complaint for a typical patient was boredom.

For scleroderma, the new CAST regimen had turned the most difficult autoimmune disease to transplant into one of the easiest. I always worried about a scleroderma patient going to the intensive care unit (MICU). The old days when I was trained at Johns Hopkins and Fred Hutchinson in a dedicated bone marrow transplant critical care unit had vanished. In the hospital I was at, HSCT was performed on a general nursing floor with nurses trained to give chemotherapy and care for central lines. Beyond that, the nurses were instructed to transfer the patient to the MICU at the first sign of instability. Patients with scleroderma often have at baseline a low blood pressure and rapid heart rate. Unless understood *a priori* that a scleroderma patient may at baseline have low blood pressure, upon standing hospital orders, the nurse would call a rapid response team who, not being familiar with the patient or this rare disease, may inappropriately push fluids or start vasopressors, exacerbating cardiopulmonary (heart/lung) compromise.

The Johns Hopkins days of the same attending physician spending at least one month on service and often sleeping those nights next to the unit had also vanished. The MICU attending physician rotated out every two weeks, and every weekend there was often another different weekend attending physician on shift. I continued rounding on the patients and did my best to influence care, but I had no authority to write orders or call the shots. Continuity of care was lost, and that always made me nervous.

Sometimes this lack of continuity in care became ridiculous. In one instance, a patient undergoing HSCT was transferred to the MICU by the night hospitalist because the patient's heart rate and rhythm had become abnormal. The MICU had a technician perform a relatively expensive heart ultrasound study (echocardiogram) and started various continuous infusion intravenous heart rhythm drugs that were intended to, but did not, slow her heart rate.

I suspected that the central line in her arm (called a PICC) had slipped forward into the heart. The line was irritating the inside of the heart, causing the irregular heart rate. This just required a noninvasive portable chest radiograph (X-ray) to confirm the position of the central catheter. After requesting an X-ray that confirmed the catheter was inside her heart chamber, we were told that the intensive care unit (ICU) could not pull the catheter back and would have to consult vascular surgery to do it. My nurse and I were flabbergasted. If the patient had remained on my service, we would have pulled the line back ourselves. Without me saying anything, my nurse walked into the MICU room, cut the stitches, and pulled the central line (PICC) back one inch. The patient's heart rhythm and rate immediately returned to normal, and she was transferred back to my service.

One saving grace was that I worked with an extremely hardworking, bright, and dedicated cardiologist who understood scleroderma. We were on the same page. When he was available, we would tag-team the ICU. (There are several types of intensive care units, such as medical or surgical.) The ICU attendings are very bright, competent, compassionate, and well-trained. It was the system that minimized continuity of care and placed a large, generalized ICU in charge of two very specialized areas (transplants and scleroderma) that had been rarely seen together.

I admired the organ (kidney, liver, intestine, and lung) transplant physicians who were somehow able to remain the attending of record on their patients when they are transferred to the surgical intensive care unit (SICU). That seemingly commonsense approach was not afforded to or fought for by the medical attendings.

Fortunately, the CAST regimen markedly decreased the risk of transfer to the MICU even for scleroderma patients with bad hearts. CAST lifted a heavy weight off my shoulders, and the short-term outcome with CAST (fludarabine, Cytoxan 60 mg/kg, ATG, rituximab) appears to be as good as the results from the ASSIST (Cytoxan 200mg/kg, ATG) regimen. A physician cannot change institutional support or lack of it, but for HSCT, you can change your conditioning regimen or patient selection.

Special Forces

At age twelve, he was in uniform in a military academy. He remained in uniform his entire life—that is, until scleroderma stripped him of his uniform. He had been trained to fight through extreme physical and mental circumstances. He rose through the officer ranks to that of major within the US Army Special Forces known as the Green Berets.

Major Cook was a Ranger Qualified, Special Forces Green Beret officer. He was involved in multiple overseas operations around the globe, including operations in South America, Central America, Iraq, and Afghanistan. He was mentally focused to accomplish tactical- and strategic-level operations and physically trained to an elite athlete status. He stood six feet, two inches tall and was 240 pounds of well-defined, ripped muscle with only 6 percent body fat. Special Forces training took him to the limits of mind and body and then pushed him beyond even that.

The men he commanded were all type A and psychologically identical to him. The opportunity to lead them was his life's most amazing and unforgettable experience. Major Cook once told me, "In battle, you are all equal." In some Romance languages (Portuguese, Spanish, Italian) the word for war is *guerra*. It is derived from a Germanic word used by Germanic tribes who invaded the Roman Empire and means *chaos*. War is total chaos. You depend on your men as much as they do on you. Knowing that you could be dead in a second, and that you are entirely dependent on one another to stay alive during moments of total chaos, forever changes the passage of time and how one interprets reality. You only really live life when you face death. Surviving a hellish, chaotic battle together is a bond sealed in blood.

Major Cook survived multiple battles, sometimes barely. While conducting night patrol in enemy-held mountainous terrain, he and a portion of his team came under enemy fire. During maneuvers, he fell down a very steep mountainside before stopping at the bottom with multiple internal and external injuries. However, the enemy had been engaged and the situation was neutralized with no one else on his team wounded—all in all, a good day. The motto of the Special Forces is De Oppresso Liber (To Free the Oppressed). They "Never Quit." Green Berets accept physically and mentally demanding assignments without complaint until retirement, death, or their medical officer orders "enough." They do not quit on their own.

The medical order of "enough" came when Major Cook was diagnosed with scleroderma. He was now facing a new battle with a stealth enemy that he had to face alone without his regiment. This was an enemy that had stripped him of his command and his rank and absolutely would never quit.

At the end of a sunny North Carolina day, his forearm looked sunburned with a gridlike alligator skin pattern. He tried aloe vera lotion, but the alligator-like hide spread and tightness around his joints started. A week later, a rheumatologist diagnosed him with scleroderma. Progression of the disease happened rapidly. Lethargy set in. Both arms became constricted and frozen up to his shoulders.

Every week he experienced a noticeable deterioration, visibly and in decreased movements. His quality of life deteriorated monthly, if not weekly. His chest, stomach, arms, and right quadriceps had the consistency of coarse leather, hard and not pliable. When walking less than one hundred yards, he had to stop and rest due to shortness of breath and muscle aches. His hands that had always been so reliable in self-defense, whether using a weapon or practicing martial arts, became dysfunctional. They would not move or bend. Even the smallest manipulations became impossible. Now even doing daily acts of self-care such as shaving or buttoning a shirt were impossible. His wife took charge of those tasks. Driving was an impossibility due to arm and hand tightness and joint contractures. His legs lost the strength to lift his body. His wife had to dress him.

Major Cook's weight dropped from 240 pounds of pure muscle to 170 pounds without any strength. Looking into the mirror and seeing his body was like looking at a stranger. It took a toll on his mental health. He knew he was in trouble and trapped. Every morning in his mind, he used his Special Forces training to prepare for that day. Each day, he repeated to himself, "It could always be worse. Hold your position and never quit. No man will be left behind." These words would snap back his will to live. But scleroderma tightened its hold. His heart and kidneys began shutting down. His skin was pulled so tightly across his stomach that a needle would not penetrate it. The steel needle bent without drawing blood or even piercing the skin.

All this had transpired within one year before Major Cook arrived for HSCT. A Green Beret Chief Warrant Officer (CWO), "Chief," who had been under his command accompanied him to clinic. I did not say anything, but I was struck by their trust and bond. They had a friendship that would have been nonexistent in the egotistical ivory tower of academic medicine. I was struck how these two Green Berets—a major and a CWO—intuitively accepted me to take command. He was in a fight for his life, which he was losing without an opportunity to fight back. Though he had decades of military training and had fought live battles behind enemy lines, he trusted me to take command, even though I was a civilian and my only quasi-military experience was as a former lieutenant commander in the US Public Health Service.

I read Major Cook and his friend the riot act of complications that may arise from transplant, including death. It did not faze either of them. They had faced death many times. What they had never faced before was having no plan to fight back. In military jargon, they were "black on." Only they were not just running low on resources—they had no resources. They knew that I had a plan, and they were ready to follow. Not to fight back, not to know how to fight back, was not acceptable.

Despite Major Cook having a disease-compromised heart, I approved his transplant in the spring of 2019 using my new CAST heart-safe regimen. The process was uneventful.

Major Cook had lost the ability to lift his body. He mostly just laid in bed during the transplant hospitalization. Seven days after stem cell infusion, while still in the hospital, he awoke one morning and was able to lift his body and move his hip. For the previous eight months, he had been unable to make those movements. His face lit up. From that day on, he knew the tide of battle had, for the first time in a year, swung to his side. He had finally broken out of scleroderma's constricting encirclement.

Over time, the skin on his face began to loosen. His heart and kidneys started working much better. His 100-meter-long walk gradually improved to a mile-long walk. At eighteen months post-transplant, he started playing ice hockey with disabled veterans on the Carolina Warriors, a team from the USA Hockey League. He joined a gym and began working on cardio exercises.

Without any new immune drugs since transplant and now two years post-HSCT, Major Cook's weight is back up to 215 pounds, and he is physically able to do basically whatever he wants. His arms have not relaxed completely, but they continue to gradually release. His stomach still has some tightness but is 95 percent back to normal. The skin on his right leg (right quad) has released and returned to normal, and his skin pigmentation is now its usual color. Opening his mouth has improved to 65 percent of normal at this time. The only residual symptoms not improving are his Raynaud's syndrome and some digital calcification that resulted in a partial thumb amputation.

Major Cook is not just courageous and intelligent, he is philosophical and reflective. He has no regrets or bitterness. As he told me two years after receiving HSCT, "My story has many highs and lows, but in the end all things work as they are supposed to. People and events enter and leave your life for many reasons; while most are forgotten or merely a footnote, a few special people have an enduring positive impact in one's life." I have remembered his words and taken them to heart during my own tough times.

Major Cook is now a retired Green Beret. He is founder and CEO of his own company. A current US congressman has been encouraging him to run for the US Congress. I hope he does.

Reincarnation

Ming used to join her husband, Kyle, on medical missions throughout the world. Her scleroderma started seven years before HSCT. When she came for evaluation, she was in a wheelchair, had lost the ability to button her clothes, could barely feed herself, and had lost function of her arms and legs. Shortness of breath was a problem with any type of exertion. She was unable to work and needed help to get to the bathroom.

Now three and a half years post HSCT, Ming functions normally, cooking, cleaning, and, as Kyle said, "She exercises like a maniac." He has his wife back. Ming received the CAST heart-safe regimen. Her only post-HSCT complications were Graves thyroid disease and low platelet counts. I added rituximab to her post-HSCT regimen, and after four weekly outpatient rounds, her platelets normalized with no further therapy. (We now routinely give rituximab with the CAST regimen.) Ming's scleroderma has disappeared. As soon as COVID permits, she and her husband are planning a return to medical mission work. Ming told my nurse that she believes in reincarnation and that HSCT had reincarnated her.

Kyle is a physician who started mountain climbing as an undergraduate at Dartmouth College. After graduating from medical school, he and his best friend, Jack, who had just graduated from law school, decided to climb as high as they could on the Tibetan side of Mount Everest, without climbing gear or tent, traveling with pilgrims and nomads like adventurers a hundred years ago. It was their last carefree adventure of youth.

With simple backpacks and wearing sneakers, they reached twenty-two thousand feet, the same altitude as the highest peak in the Western Hemisphere, Cerro Aconcagua in the Andes. At that altitude, facing bitter cold, suffering frostbitten extremities, and having no oxygen, they decided they had accomplished their goal. By law, all planes must have the cabin pressurized with oxygen when above 14,000 feet. They were hiking at 22,000 feet without oxygen. Kyle had lost over 40 pounds.

They were ready to return to civilization for a shower and some cold beers in Lhasa, the capital of Tibet. The world was theirs. For many people, it is often unclear when exactly one enters adulthood. For them, it happened in an instant when their youthful innocence was stripped away. Like a twilight zone door to an alternate universe, the world they came back to was not the same world they had left before trekking to Mount Everest.

Kyle and Jack hitchhiked to Lhasa with stickers of the Tibetan flag on their backpacks. Chinese police arrested them at gunpoint and interrogated them for days. The Chinese do not provide a defense lawyer or allow silence to prevent inadvertent self-incrimination. Kyle and Jack avoided reacting defensively to allegations and calmly and consistently answered questions that were repeatedly voiced as accusations. There were threats of transporting them to a prison in Beijing for more "refined" interrogation techniques if they did not admit to some sort of wrongdoing. Their offense: having the Tibetan flag on their backpacks.

American citizenship afforded them some protection that Tibetans did not have, as the Chinese Central Committee did not wish to transfer them to Beijing and risk possible escalation to an international incident. After several days, they were released and given their passports back. They were told to tell the world that the Chinese were improving the lives of Tibetans. To this day, they have done exactly the opposite. They were and are 100 percent with the Tibetans.

Lhasa was in crisis. Tibetans were demonstrating after Tibetan monks had been beaten. The Chinese police paraded a truckload of Tibetans through the streets with loudspeakers blaring. In a public execution, they tied their hands, broke their elbows and ribs so they could not shout "Free Tibet," and then shot them in the back of the head. Each executed prisoner's family was forced to pay the police the equivalent of five dollars for the cost of the bullet. Buddhist temples were raided, trashed, and set on fire. Police opened fire with AK-47s, killing men, women, and children. Under the pretense of overpopulation, Tibetan woman were forcibly sterilized to prevent them from having more children. Tibet has fewer people per square mile than Australia.

Physicians and staff performed these forced abortions in Chinese government run "Peoples' Hospitals." During my training, physicians were taught that no medical professional, including no physician, can treat a patient without a patient's consent (except in an emergency when the patient or next of kin cannot speak for themselves). I was taught that to operate on or medicate a person without their consent is considered assault. For myself, the entire foundation of Western law, including how I practice medicine, is based on the principle of consent. The difference between a gift and theft is consent. The difference between making love and rape is consent. The difference between giving a medication or doing surgery and assaulting a patient is consent.

Kyle tried, as best he could with no medical supplies, to treat wounded Tibetan civilians in the street. A ten-year-old boy died in his hands from a Chinese bullet to the heart. They witnessed eleven deaths in one day. All were either shot or beaten to death with shovels. Kyle traveled at night by rooftop to treat the wounded.

Kyle and Jack were eventually able to escape and met with the Dalai Lama in India. They told him of the crimes they had witnessed and brought him empty bullet cartridges that had been fired at Tibetans. The spiritual leader of Buddhism absorbed everything. Before departing, the Dalai Lama thanked them for their compassion and courage and then calmly said, "Most people bring me flowers. You are the first to bring me bullets."

Back in America, Kyle and Jack told their story in interviews on television and radio and in newspapers and to a congressional committee, but without proof, nobody took them seriously. So over seven different times in thirteen years, they returned separately to Tibet with hidden cameras to obtain video proof of China's prisons in Tibet. Kyle also documented China's National Family Planning Policy of coerced abortion, sterilization, and infanticide at twenty People's Hospitals in Lhasa and remote regions.

Back in America, Kyle got no traction. He turned to Europe and asked if he could present his evidence to Spain's international court on crimes against humanity. The Spanish National Court agreed, but the US Department of State objected and blocked Kyle from traveling to Spain for seven years. Without evidence, the case remained dormant.

In 2011, Kyle found a way to Madrid. He presented forty-five pounds of audio, film, and video footage to the Spanish court. The Chinese president and other Chinese leaders were found guilty of "genocide, crimes against humanity, torture, and forced disappearance and arbitrary executions." Interpol arrest warrants were issued. Behind closed doors, the American government pressured the Spanish government that subsequently revoked the court's authority to prosecute leaders of foreigner governments. The Interpol arrest warrants were rescinded.

In Tibet, Buddhism has been sidelined. The Tibetan language is not allowed to be taught in schools, and emigrant Chinese now outnumber native Tibetans. Kyle made a film that was shown at the Madrid International Film Festival and Berlin International Filmmaker Festival of World Cinema. He was nominated as "Best Director for a Short Documentary" and awarded the "Scientific and Education Award." He published a book called *Sky Burial* and released a film called *Eye of the Lammergeier*, both named out of respect for a traditional Tibetan burial custom. The film can be viewed online at: http://www.eyeofthelammergeier.com.

I have spoken about hematopoietic stem cell transplantation for autoimmune disease many times in China and, because of my talks, Chinese physicians have started using stem cells to treat patients with autoimmune diseases. The Chinese people are wonderful, kind, generous, hardworking, intelligent, gracious, respectful, and very family oriented. When the COVID pandemic first struck, its virulence was unknown and there were few N-95 face masks available in America to protect people from the virus. Without asking, a physician in China shipped me two large boxes of N-95 masks that I distributed among staff and patients. Unlike America, big cities in China are very safe to walk around in. Newspaper and Internet discourse are refreshingly polite and respectful without the personal attack-oriented commentary that is so common in America.

The question often asked after atrocities is how a cultured people can do such things. The Army is not a democracy. Its cohesiveness and effectiveness depend on obeying orders. The psychological pressure to do as you are told is understood when you enlist. But how can educated, well trained, thoughtful physicians in modern medical institutions participate in forced sterilizations? Is pressure to conform a potential side effect inherent to all institutions? Massachusetts Institutes of Technology Professor Noam Chomsky commented about educational institutions: "The whole educational and professional training system is a very elaborate filter, which just weeds out people who are too independent, and who think for themselves, and who don't know how to be submissive, and so on—because they're dysfunctional to the institutions."

Years later, I was invited to the Chinese embassy for a ceremony. I was an out-of-place doctor surrounded by various foreign embassy diplomats. Because I thought it would be interesting and educational, I brought along my son, who was in high school at the time. When the Chinese consulate offered a toast from the stage, my son, who had never heard Ming and Kyle's story (nor any patient's story) turned to me and said out loud, "Is now the time to shout *Free Tibet*?" Diplomats standing around us turned around in shock and disbelief. Who had allowed such Neanderthal troglodytes into this event? Out of respect for my Chinese hosts, because I do not like public scenes, and because this was not the time or place for such a comment, I hushed my son. But he was right, and I am proud of him.

Today Ming and Kyle are planning a medical mission to Southeast Asia. She is the "boots on the ground" of their medical work. She speaks multiple Asian languages and several hill tribe dialects. They are both barred from ever returning to Tibet or China, nor would I want them to take that personal risk.

The Scleroderma Gut

As mentioned throughout this chapter, scleroderma affects the skin, lungs, heart, and kidneys. It also affects the gastrointestinal tract (gut). One potentially dangerous complication of scleroderma is gastric antral vascular ectasia (GAVE), also called "watermelon stomach." GAVE is specific to scleroderma (it is not found in multiple sclerosis). Remember that scleroderma is an immune-mediated vasculopathy (a small blood vessel disease). GAVE is a fancy term for disordered and malformed (telangiectasia) blood vessels in the stomach. GAVE vessels will intermittently and asymptomatically ooze blood, causing iron-deficiency anemia. It is a hidden, occult, low-grade bleed that almost never causes gross blood in the stool or black stool (blood, when digested, turns black and tarry). At least, patients do not notice it or complain of it.

GAVE is common in scleroderma patients with iron-deficiency anemia (picked up on routine blood counts) or telangiectasias of the skin that are commonly found on the face. These can be overlooked during a cursory exam, as it is common for female scleroderma patients to heroically cover up twisted facial blood vessels (telangiectasias) with makeup.

The HSCT conditioning regimen temporarily lowers a patient's platelet (cells that clot blood) count. Until recovery of the patient's platelets that varies from five to ten days depending upon conditioning regimen, GAVE in the stomach may suddenly switch from a low, intermittent, asymptomatic bleed to a life-threatening waterfall of blood (hemorrhage) due to this low platelet count. Trial by fire taught me that pre-HSCT any scleroderma patient with anemia or telangiectasias needed to have an endoscopy and if GAVE is present, even if not bleeding, must be treated with laser cauterization. Cauterization prevents future bleeding by burning the blood vessels closed.

Many gastroenterologists are unaware of the risk of a serious HSCT-induced GAVE bleed. When putting a scope in a scleroderma patient's stomach, GAVE is almost always not bleeding at that moment in time. Without any active bleeding present at that moment, many gastroenterologists routinely refuse to cauterize the blood vessels. Despite explaining why cauterization is necessary, I have had far too many GI doctors refuse to perform cauterization. When I persist, they usually tell me to find someone else. And that is the key—to find a GI doctor who understands HSCT and why GAVE, even when the patient is not bleeding at that moment, needs cauterization before undergoing HSCT. When you connect with such a gastroenterologist, it's just like working with the right scleroderma cardiologist (heart doctor)—they are worth their weight in gold. Unfortunately, there is a growing tendency for hospitals to insist that you work with whoever is working for the hospital and is on call at that moment. It is a paperwork mentality of checking the box to fill an "employee" position, which rotates you around the merry-go-round back to where you started.

The Model and the Hulk

Judy is a medical doctor of dentistry. She is a tall, beautiful, intelligent woman who trained and taught at Rutgers University. As a Rutgers student, she met and married her husband, who now works as a Rutgers security guard and is built like a combination of Lou Ferrigno and Mr. T. He is also as kind, soft-spoken, and as gentle as the Hulk's counterpart, Robert Bruce Banner.

At the time of HSCT, Judy had scleroderma for three years, and already had survived a prior scleroderma renal (kidney) crisis. Her entire body (except her back) was turning rock-hard, including her arms, hands, legs, abdomen, and chest. She could not get out of a chair, became short of breath when walking with assistance a few feet, and was wheelchair-dependent.

During the transplant, Judy started to bleed from GAVE in her stomach. At first, we managed her on the floor with drugs to decrease stomach acid, transfusions of blood, and frequent checks of her cell counts. As transfusion requirements increased, she was transferred to the MICU.

This was an instance where the transfer was happening as it should: seamless and all caregivers functioning as a team. As Judy's transfusion requirements increased, upon my request the blood bank moved a blood component refrigerator loaded with blood products into her MICU room. This prevented a time delay from ordering, preparing, and transporting blood products. I asked gastroenterology services to put a scope into her stomach to evaluate and stop the bleeding with laser cauterization. Because the bleeding had become so profuse, she needed to be sedated and intubated.

I had stepped away to another floor and received an urgent page to return to Judy's room. I literally ran back to the unit. A little short of breath, I held her hand and told her to accept the sedation and intubation, not just to allow a machine to breathe for her but also to protect her airway so that the blood from her stomach would not flood up into her lungs. I saw the apprehension in her eyes. The thought of being put to sleep and possibly never awakening, along with trusting another person to bring you back, is scary. But Judy knew what she had to do. I felt her draw from a well of courage deep inside her.

We sedated and intubated her and when the GI doctor inserted a scope into her, I watched on a digital screen and looked directly through the scope. The hope for a quick fix evaporated. There was no single vessel to shut off. GAVE is a mess of microscopic vessels just under the mucosa (first layer of the stomach) that oozes blood from every direction. As soon as water was squirted onto a part of her stomach to wash away the blood, more blood immediately seeped out from every direction. It was like the stomach wall itself had become a porous membrane. Blood was spilling forth like liquid through a kitchen strainer. Severe bleeding depletes proteins that clot blood, which further worsens bleeding. Surgery of any kind would have caused more unstoppable bleeding.

Fresh frozen plasma (blood clotting proteins), cryoprecipitate (a concentrated form of blood clotting proteins), platelet transfusions (cells to clot blood), and red blood cells (cells to transport oxygen) had to be continuously infused through three different central line catheters. As soon as one bag was infused, another was pulled from the refrigerator next to Judy's bed and immediately hung. The nurses were focused, efficient, and on top of everything. Unit nurses are on the front line and, by training, immediately run to help any other nurse who is becoming overwhelmed. They worked together as if one mind were controlling their bodies. Together, they supported Judy through a massive hemorrhage. I swore to myself that I would never let this happen to another patient. Patients will have GAVE cauterized before the transplant! Her husband, a massive hulk of a man who could stop an M-1 Abrams battle tank, remained calm, polite, and gentle throughout it all. Although I have seen it with every patient, I am amazed by the unconditional faith a seriously ill patient and their family entrust to you.

Judy is now seven years post-HSCT and can walk up and down stairs and drive a car. She has no shortness of breath, and most of her joint contractures have disappeared. Her heart and kidneys, which had been damaged by scleroderma, are functioning well. She has had no further gut bleeding. Her hand contractures have improved, but limitation of finger fine motion prevents practicing dentistry. Judy's recovery was also facilitated by a dedicated local nephrologist (kidney doctor) who was always available, on top of Judy's care, and easy to work with.

Because of this experience, before HSCT every patient of mine with anemia or telangiectasia receives endoscopy and laser cauterization. No clinical GAVE bleed during transplant has happened since.

Scleroderma also commonly causes a wide-open esophagus (the muscular tube that connects the mouth to the stomach), termed a *patulous esophagus*. In order to document recovery of esophageal muscle strength, a tube with an inflatable balloon can be placed in the esophagus to measure pressure from muscle contractions (manometry).

After the first few patients reported the same visceral dislike for this common GI test, I stopped doing it. The scientific answer was not worth the discomfort to my patients. Although all knowledge is potentially beneficial, knowing that information would not directly change patient care or detract from the benefits of HSCT.

Beyond GAVE or a patulous (gaping open) esophagus, scleroderma may in some cases cause severe gastrointestinal malabsorption (poor absorption of nutrients) and slow transit or stasis of food in the gut.

Returning to Law School

While in law school on the East Coast, Cheyanne developed severe skin and gut scleroderma. She was unable to walk, confined to a wheelchair, and unable to transfer to the toilet (transfer is medical jargon for ability to move from one surface to another) without assistance. Her weight dropped from 205 pounds to 88 pounds. Attempts to eat caused prolonged nausea and repeated vomiting. She survived on total parenteral nutrition (TPN), which is the liquid infusion of proteins, fats, and minerals into the veins. Scleroderma had caused Cheyanne's intestines to stop functioning. From experience, I knew that her skin and mobility, as horrific as it was, would get better after HSCT, but I did not know if her gut would improve. Despite the unknowns, she wanted the transplant.

Her transplant was in 2008. Small improvements in her skin began immediately, but her gut showed no immediate signs of regaining function. After transplant, Cheyanne was transferred to rehabilitation. She remained in rehab and on TPN for six months. I was concerned that her gut may never improve, but around six months after HSCT, it started to regain function. Improvement was initially in baby steps, but by one year, she was permanently off TPN, eating food and drinking liquids without nausea or vomiting, and walking without assistance. She returned to law school and completed her law degree.

Cheyanne passed the bar exam and is now in practice. She bought a house and is engaged. Cheyanne can now do everything a typical person can do, except she still has trouble putting on a sock or squatting, and about every two years she undergoes esophageal dilation as an outpatient. She eats normally, returned to a normal weight, drives, and works full time as a lawyer. Perhaps her most exceptional trait is that throughout all of this, she has always remained a very positive-energy person whose optimism and love for life and other people have never faded. She always finds the best in every person.

Results of Other Randomized Trials for HSCT and Scleroderma

HSCT is now accepted as a standard treatment for systemic sclerosis and is routinely paid for by insurance companies. Three randomized trials have demonstrated the superiority of HSCT over the traditional standard of care.

Two trials were nonmyeloablative. My American ASSIST trial, published in *The Lancet* (2011 and 2013) and the European ASTIS (2014) trial, published in *JAMA*, used almost identical regimens of Cytoxan and ATG and demonstrated the superiority of HSCT. The European ASTIS used a higher dose of ATG (7.5 mg/kg) and removal of immune cells from the reinfused hematopoietic (blood) stem cells (called CD34 selection). It was associated with a viral (Epstein-Barr virus, EBV) death. ASSIST had no EBV infections or viral deaths due to a lower total dose of ATG (6.0 mg/kg) and use of an unmanipulated (no selection outside the body) autologous hematopoietic stem cell graft.

The important point is that more aggressive immune ablation, even with a nonmyeloablative regimen, is not necessarily better. The goal is to achieve immune tolerance with minimal risk of infections and toxicity to the patient. Outcomes from the Cytoxan/ATG studies (ASSIST and ASTIS) were significantly better compared to the standard of care control arm. There were marked improvements in skin, lung, quality of life, and survival.

The third trial was the myeloablative total body irradiation NIAID trial called SCOT. It was not reported until 2018.[9] It had the smallest number of transplant patients (thirty-three treated with HSCT) due to difficulty in attracting and enrolling patients. As mentioned earlier, patients did not want to enroll for two reasons: they did not want the risk of cancer from total body irradiation, and they wanted to cross over to HSCT if the control arm failed, but that would have been prohibited according to the terms of the SCOT trial. I was the only physician to walk away from the SCOT trial. In my mind, a physician's priority is always to do what is best for their patient.

In the SCOT trial with total body irradiation, the lung function did not improve and 9 percent of the HSCT survivors (at the time of publication) developed radiation-induced cancers: two myelodysplastic leukemias and one thyroid (medullary) tumor. The problem with total body irradiation-induced cancer is that the incidence of new radiation-induced cancers will keep increasing even more throughout the patient's remaining life span.

The study end point in SCOT changed during the middle of the study. They changed from a hard end point of survival to a mathematically averaged end point that combined many different end points into one final score. From an ethics standpoint, one should not change the primary end point in the middle of a study. It allows the investigator (consciously or unconsciously) to insert bias into the data analysis and interpretation. The investigators are, in effect, allowed to interpret data in the middle of trial to redirect the ending of the story.[10] This can be ethically done if the ongoing results are unknown by those changing the end point,[11] but in reality, the motivation to

Study Name	Conditioning regimen	Stem cell CD34 select	HSCT Improved skin and QOL	Better lung function after HSCT	Shown to cause cancer	Days of low blood counts	Move to ICU during HSCT	Cost of HSCT
CAST	Nonmyeloablative Fludarabine, Cytoxan ATG, Rituxan	No	Yes	Yes	No	5	No	+ Lowest cost
ASSIST	Nonmyeloablative Cytoxan ATG	No	Yes	Yes	No	9-10	Rare	++
ASTIS	Nonmyeloablative Cytoxan ATG	Yes	Yes	Yes	No	9-10	Minor	++
SCOT	Myeloablative Total body irradiation Cytoxan ATG	Yes	Yes	No	Yes	9-10	More common	+++ Highest cost

Table 5. Differences between hematopoietic stem cell transplant (HSCT) trials for scleroderma. ATG = antithymocyte globulin, CD34 = a marker on hematopoietic stem cells, Cytoxan = cyclophosphamide, ICU = intensive care unit, QOL = quality of life, TBI = total body irradiation. Trial names CAST = cardiac safe transplant, ASSIST = American scleroderma stem cell versus immune suppression trial, ASTIS = Autologous stem cell transplant immune suppression trial, SCOT = scleroderma, cyclophosphamide or transplant.

change the end point is often *a priori* knowledge that the primary end point is failing.

The differences between CAST, ASSIST, ASTIS and SCOT are shown in Table 5.

As my Special Forces Green Beret patient said about his own experience, "In the end everything works out as it should." Outside of America, especially in Europe, Mexico, Brazil, and Asia, the less expensive, nonmyeloablative, non-radiation regimen (ASSIST or ASTIS) is the standard. More recently, several international centers (France, Israel, Norway) have been switching to the even safer and cheaper nonmyeloablative CAST regimen. The common-sense future, even in America, will be toward using safer, less expensive regimens.

While I did not know how to help her at the time, I finally know what to do for the seventeen-year-old girl with shortness of breath whose hand I held and whose green eyes looked into mine at 2:00 in the morning during my first year of internship fresh out of medical school. As the French novelist Victor Hugo said, "Nothing is more powerful than an idea whose time has come."

CHAPTER 6

NEUROMYELITIS OPTICA (NMO): CONFUSED WITH MS

Most conscientious speakers prepare their lectures well in advance. I did it the night before, during the trip, or upon arrival, which I would not, in general, advise. However, I pioneered the HSCT field and had plenty to speak about from my own patient care experience, as I made myself available 24/7 at my patients' bedsides. As the colloquialism goes, I knew HSCT like the back of my hand and did not necessarily need the time for prepping. At one event, I spoke about HSCT for multiple sclerosis and shared the cab fare back to the airport with a physician from the Mayo Clinic.

Academics may at times be pompous and guarded, which is in part out of paranoid insecurity that someone else will pilfer your idea and publish before you, as has happened to virtually everyone in academics at one time or another. My taxi co-share was, on the contrary, very open and unguarded. He was a breath of fresh air. During that cab ride, he explained neuromyelitis optica (NMO), a rare immune-mediated demyelinating disease of the brain and spinal cord that I had barely even heard of before. He suggested that HSCT might be an effective treatment for the disease.

Because of a busy schedule, it took me time to learn about the disease and develop a protocol for treating it. I began, like always, intermittently reading anything I could on NMO. I soon recognized that the Mayo Clinic was a leading center for NMO. Their group discovered an antibody that is diagnostic for the disease and defined the criteria for diagnosis of NMO. The antibody, called aquaporin 4 (AQP4), targets astrocytes (nurse or support cells) within the central nervous system and, in general, the higher the titer (level) of AQP4 antibody, the greater the likelihood of a severe clinical attack. Identifying this antibody was no small accomplishment because most autoimmune diseases do not have a biological marker.

NMO is commonly confused with multiple sclerosis. Like multiple sclerosis, it is a central nervous system demyelinating disease, but it is not multiple sclerosis. NMO may be differentiated from multiple sclerosis by the presence of the AQP4 antibody and predominant involvement of optic nerves and long lesions within the spinal cord. The magnetic resonance imaging (MRI) appearance shows lesions in the spine that are continuous (no interruption) for at least three vertebral bodies in length. There are seven cervical and twelve thoracic vertebrae in the human body. A lesion that spans three or more vertebrae in length is extensive. In contrast, the spinal lesions in multiple sclerosis are usually less than one vertebra in length. Traditionally, the prognosis for NMO is that 50 percent of patients will have trouble walking or be legally blind within five years of diagnosis.

The nonmyeloablative conditioning regimen I selected for NMO was plasmapheresis, Cytoxan, ATG, and rituximab.[1] Cytoxan is an immune cell-specific chemotherapy. ATG and rituximab are proteins (antibodies) directed against immune cells. Plasmapheresis is a technique of removing the plasma from the blood. Plasma is 92 percent salt water; the other 8 percent is composed of mostly fats, sugars, minerals, vitamins, hormones, and proteins, including antibodies such as anti-AQP4 that causes NMO. The goal of plasmapheresis is to temporally decrease the anti-AQP4 antibodies.

I chose this regimen because once I had a patient with "multiple sclerosis" undergo HSCT with my usual Cytoxan and ATG conditioning regimen who relapsed early after transplant with a severe attack. The early relapse and location of the relapse were very unusual after HSCT of multiple sclerosis, and a one-off from my clinical experience. A repeat diagnostic workup revealed that the patient really had NMO. The conditioning regimen of Cytoxan and ATG was not strong enough for neuromyelitis optica. While this was a one-of-a-kind experience that nobody would consider definitive, it was the index case or primer that made me add plasmapheresis and rituximab, an antibody that targets immune B cells, to my NMO regimen. The AQP4 antibodies are made by B cells. It was still a nonmyeloablative regimen, and the patient's bone marrow and blood counts would recover even without reinfusion of stem cells.

The Basketball Game

Fred was the first patient who underwent HSCT for the diagnosis of NMO. He came from the West Coast and had been originally incorrectly diagnosed with multiple sclerosis by neurologists in California. Fred's disease began with an attack of optic neuritis manifested as blurred vision in both eyes, making it impossible for him to read. He was treated with steroids. A few months later, optic neuritis recurred, and he was treated this time with steroids and intravenous immunoglobulins (IVIG) which caused headaches and nausea for days after each infusion. On his third attack, he was hospitalized with paralysis on his left side from the waist down. He went home using a walker and started taking more anti-multiple sclerosis drugs chronically. These drugs made him feel worse, so against doctor's advice, he terminated the multiple sclerosis drugs. This was fortuitous because some multiple sclerosis drugs make NMO worse. It is unfortunately relatively common for NMO to be misdiagnosed as multiple sclerosis.

Within two years from exhibiting his first symptom, Fred suffered a fourth attack. He was again hospitalized, could not swallow food, went into a coma for about ten days, and was treated with steroids, plasmapheresis, and rituximab (an anti-B immune cell drug).

Upon awaking, Fred was paralyzed from the neck down, and a feeding tube had been inserted into his nose. After a month in a rehabilitation facility, he was able to use a wheelchair. He went home in the wheelchair. His wife, daughter, and son installed ramps at the entry of their home and took the doors off every room in the house, including the bedrooms and the bathroom, so he could enter them in his wheelchair.

After two years of treatments, the venomous AQP4 antibody remained in his blood, and he remained wheelchair-bound. Medical care was not working, and Fred was headed toward hospice care or death with his next attack. At this point, Fred asked his daughter to search the Internet for anything that she could find on NMO. She found our clinical stem cell trial.

Since this was the first time performing HSCT for NMO, I was concerned that it may not work. If this was multiple sclerosis, after being in a wheelchair for one year, it would have been called progressive MS, and I had enough data by then to know a transplant would not reverse the deficits from progressive MS. But I knew that every disease is different, and although Fred was in a wheelchair, he could use a walker to travel at least a few steps.

When playing poker against NMO, HSCT turned out to be the royal flush. Before being discharged after HSCT, Fred could eat without throwing up, and his disabling chronic hiccups were gone. Returning to his own home, he got stronger every day. Within one month, he was able to walk with a cane, within two months was able to walk on his own without the cane or any device for assistance, and within six months he was riding a bicycle, doing yard work, and driving a car again.

At six months after HSCT, Fred sent me a video of himself riding a bicycle in the street and shooting basketball hoops in his driveway. It had been years since he could jump off the ground. The basketball swished through the hoop without even hitting the rim. I heard his wife cheering in the background. But this was not just some regular basketball game over who gets the most points. That basketball swish meant Fred had won his life back. And in my mind, he had just bested Michael Jordan.

At the time of writing this chapter, it has been eleven years since his transplant. During this time, Fred has been on no medications and has had no attacks and no new or worsening symptoms. His wife no longer needs to be his care provider. She returned to working full time. Today Fred has a normal life. Now in retirement, he is fixing up his current home and is real estate shopping to buy a new house in a location where he hopes to enjoy more open outdoor space for hiking and walking.

The Guthy-Jackson Charitable Foundation is devoted to funding research for NMO. They are a good organization and in 2010, they invited Fred and me to speak at their annual patient meeting in California. It was great to see Fred and listen to him speak on stage. Before I spoke, the moderator introduced me with the caveat that as an organization, they do not endorse any treatments, something they had not said before any other speaker took the podium.

Fred and I caught each other's eye and in that millisecond of a glance, our thoughts aligned. It was obvious that the organization was skeptical of HSCT. They were cautious because the academic neurologists who advise them tended to be conservative and skeptical. Still, they had the courage to invite both my patient and me to speak at their patient forum. New ideas begin by allowing discussion, especially when it goes against traditional thinking.

During the panel forum, patients with NMO asked how long they had to stay on medications for their NMO. Every other physician on the panel said that they should stay on medications indefinitely for fear of more frequent relapses happening when they went off treatment. Sitting at the end of the table, I was the last one to answer the question. I said that NMO patients should stop all medications after a transplant and stay off all medications indefinitely until and if a relapse occurred. The room went quiet for a short moment. Academia, for all its enlightenment, has maintained the trappings and rightness of medieval religious orthodoxy, and I had just spoken heresy.

Medicine is a conservative field, and advocates of new therapies have to prove themselves. Whenever a new treatment comes from outside the field and subspecialists in the field do not have the training to do the procedure, the burden of proof is exponentially more difficult.

As we continued treating NMO, I learned that even HSCT for NMO has its limits. Patients could be in a wheelchair and recover walking, but only if they could still at least partially lift their leg against gravity. Once dense complete paralysis sets in and persists, it's too late for HSCT to reverse the paralysis.

NCAA Basketball

Other autoimmune diseases may also coexist with NMO, such as systemic lupus erythematosus (SLE). Erica had both NMO and serologic markers for SLE and another autoimmune disease called Sjögren's syndrome. For fourteen years, her father had been the head coach of the men's basketball team for a big university. He was their all-time winningest coach and led them to several NCAA tournament appearances. Like one of the sixth century Seven Greek Sages advocating for a sound mind in a sound body, Erica was a gifted athlete and had a doctorate in educational policy.

Her first attack of NMO was a sudden loss of feeling in her left toes that ascended to her left breast. She was incorrectly diagnosed with multiple sclerosis and started on interferon without effect. After one year of interferon, she was using a wheelchair. Her diagnosis was changed to NMO and after three years of Cytoxan (cyclophosphamide), she was out of her wheelchair. She endured at least one major relapse each year, which was treated with hospitalization and intravenous corticosteroids. After an acute attack accompanied by visual loss, her diagnosis was changed to three distinct autoimmune diseases: NMO, systemic lupus erythematosus (SLE), and Sjögren's syndrome.

When referred for HSCT, Erica had been using a wheelchair for over one year. By six months post-transplant, she was walking without assistance. For the past nine years since transplant, she has never had another neurologic attack, can skip, and wears three-inch-high heels. She works full time as a chief human resources officer.

Since transplant, for the last nine years her NMO anti-AQP4 autoantibodies have remained negative. Six years after treatment, she developed a butterfly-like facial rash, patchy hair loss (alopecia), and dry eyes, symptoms consistent with systemic lupus erythematosus (SLE) and Sjögren's that now remain stable on oral medication. This is consistent with our experience for patients with SLE in that remission after HSCT for NMO lasts for decades while for SLE, 50 percent relapse within five years when using this regimen.[2] [3] Many people assume that all transplants are the same but, to the contrary, the regimens are different and need to be perfected, often through trial and error, for each different autoimmune disease. I have an idea how to improve the conditioning regimen for SLE which I have shared with creative physician researchers at Columbia but that is another story.

Brasileira (Brazilian Woman)

A woman with NMO who was in her mid-twenties emailed me from Brazil asking for help. American hospitals would not allow her to have a transplant unless her insurance company approved payment or she herself or her family paid up-front. This made the procedure impossible for most people like her, who did not have insurance.

A friend of a friend told her that I was scheduled to speak at the University of São Paulo (USP) in Ribeirão Preto, São Paulo, Brazil, about HSCT for autoimmune neurologic diseases. With bold hesitation, she asked if she could meet with me in Brazil. I was impressed by her resolve. She reminded me of myself when my fate had been in the hands of Dr. Arthur Nienhuis. As his fellow at the NIH, I had asked him if I could work on my idea of HSCT for autoimmune diseases at Johns Hopkins but remain on his NIH payroll. Dr. Nienhuis had granted my request.

I arranged to meet with my Brazilian colleagues and her at a small coffee shop in Ribeirão Preto. I guess it could be described as the longest long-distance house call ever performed. Professor Julio Voltarelli was the head of transplant at USP and our thoughts were usually on the same page. Julio agreed that maybe, in a meeting of minds, we could figure out a way to help her. In Portuguese, the expression is *dar um jeito*. The literal translation is "to give a way." The figurative meaning is to find a way to do something when the bureaucracy is against you. I knew Julio would agree to perform the transplant on her, and I would give him my protocol and experience, but I was unsure about the Brazilian neurologist. My thinking was that if he met the patient in person with Julio and me, he would find it difficult to wash his hands of the situation and walk away.

I first met Julio in San Diego after I gave Medical Grand Rounds at the University of California. He was doing a sabbatical at Scripps and came to listen to my talk. From that day forward we became friends, and Julio became an international leader in HSCT of autoimmune diseases. USP is one of the best public medical centers in Brazil, and its physicians are as good as, if not better than, any doctor in any center in America.

The young NMO Brazilian girl had traveled all night on a bus from another state to meet me. She could not speak English, but a friend who spoke some English came with her. I speak a little Portuguese, *mais ou menos* (more or less—usually less than more). I had taken three years of Latin in high school, and Brazilian Portuguese is living Latin with a few Arabic, Bantu, and native Indian words sprinkled in.

The patient had already suffered severe attacks but could still walk. When Julio arrived, he seemed to be in a bad mood, which was unusual for him. There was some animated discussion in Portuguese that was too fast for me to follow, but I gathered that there was a problem. I interrupted to ask what was wrong, and Julio told me that the neurologist had declined to meet her. I tried to speak with the neurologist, but I had no influence.

We had a treatment that could help her, but the system was working against us. Our patient remained gracious and polite, but her last hope was gone. I insisted on at least paying for her bus fare home, but she refused. She was poor, but she would not allow NMO to take her pride and dignity from her.

I have no way to know for sure, but I have little doubt that this young girl passed away long ago from NMO. Brazil has socialized, government-run "free medicine" for all citizens, but the only treatment the bureaucracy would approve for her were steroids after each attack. She could not even get plasmapheresis or intravenous immunoglobulin that were standard treatments in America.

Just like the third-grade girl standing in line at Hawthorne Elementary and the seventeen-year-old with scleroderma whom I was paged to see as a first-year resident, this young Brazilian woman's story is imprinted on my memory. In this case, I knew how to help but was stopped from helping. It is insane and inhumane. I do not want this scenario to keep repeating, especially when effective treatments exist. It is for this reason that I, along with worldwide university colleagues, wrote a medical textbook titled *Hematopoietic Stem Cell Transplantation and Cellular Therapies for Autoimmune Diseases* published in late 2021. Now I am writing this lay book, *Everyday Miracles*, because patients and their families need to know about these treatments. Patients need ammunition to help them fight the bureaucratic system. Out of memory for this Brazilian girl, I will have this book translated into Portuguese.

I was frustrated with the University of São Paulo neurologist who had said *no* to this young girl, but he was not a bad individual. Even though he was working at the Harvard of Brazil, his resources and time were limited and would have to be diverted from other projects. Academic neurology in America was also ignoring this treatment. As a neurologist, he was following the accepted norm. But one person can make a difference. The key is to see the person in front of you as a person.

Both Julio and the neurologist have now passed away. I spoke at Julio's memorial service in USP, and I brought with me a plaque signed by five US congressmen in honor of Julio's work expanding HSCT for autoimmune diseases. This plaque hangs over the BMT unit at USP.

There are problems with all systems. At USP, the hospital does not get money (is not rewarded) for doing HSCT. Instead, the hospital has a fixed government budget that must be distributed between different departments and treatments. The result is political infighting and removal of the patient (and the doctors who are not professional politicians) from deciding their own fate and treatment.

Most publications on drug treatment for NMO report one- or two-year follow-up with no data on AQP4 antibody levels. The rare report on AQP4 levels showed that it does not disappear with drug treatment. We published with five years of follow-up with AQP4 antibody levels both before and after HSCT. All patients had significant neurological improvement after HSCT. The publication only included eleven patients, but after five years two patients who remained AQP4-positive relapsed, while nine patients seroconverted to negative (the AQP4 antibody disappeared). They have remained treatment-free and disease-free for five or more years since HSCT.

The Mayo Clinic's contribution to this study was important, as AQP4 is a biomarker for disease, and the antibody levels and cell-killing assays that confirmed the clinical outcome were performed by an outside independent group (Mayo Clinic) who had no knowledge of clinical results.

Just after publication of the NMO results, I was invited to speak in Moscow, Russia. It was an international meeting, and several European colleagues who had helped to pioneer this field had been invited to speak. During the lunch break, the head of the transplant unit, Professor Denis Fedorenko, took me and Professor Dominique Farge from Paris, France, to visit transplant patients on their ward.

I was introduced to a French gentleman in his hospital bed in Moscow. He was being treated with my conditioning regimen for HSCT of NMO. He repeatedly thanked me and, in the customary French manner, hugged and kissed me on both cheeks. I did not want him exposed to my germs, but it happened too fast to prevent. He knew who had designed his treatment, and he was so sincerely grateful. It is a small world—a French national, treated in a Moscow university hospital with my conditioning regimen, speaking with a French physician about his frustration in not being able to get HSCT for NMO in France, a wealthy first-world country.

Regulatory frameworks are essential to minimize false hopes or financial exploitation of patients and to ensure safe development of new fields. Such regulations are a fundamental part of quality care. But as I left this patient's room, I felt mixed emotions—admiration for the courage of this Frenchman and frustration for the indifference, arrogance, obstacles, and slow change of entrenched bureaucracies to cope with and relieve the suffering of an individual patient.

The first drug approved (in 2019) by the FDA for NMO was eculizumab (eh-kuh-LOO-zuh-mab). It costs a patient $750,000 US dollars each year. The drug only blocks a pathway (complement activation); it does not change the underlying disease etiology. It does not get rid of the antibody that causes the disease. You remain on the drug forever, or until you experience an attack.

Rituximab is a fraction of the cost of eculizumab, and it decreases (but does not eliminate) the pathologic antibody titer, but because its patent has expired, nobody will make money from it. An American neurologist whom I very much respect and who trained in another country once said to me (before other drugs for NMO were approved), "As the only FDA-approved drug for NMO, Americans will pay $750,000 a year for eculizumab. Countries that cannot afford it can use rituximab." To me, this is a startling admission of the corrosive effect of an American system that does not reward physicians for prioritizing cost-effectiveness. If you want a problem to be accepted as normal, do not hide it, put in directly in front of people. Their eyes will remain wide closed.

What insurance company or society can afford three quarters of a million US dollars each and every year for one patient with NMO? Especially when there are more cost-effective but non-patented treatments? HSCT is a one-time treatment that costs for NMO approximately $125,000 (the conditioning regimen for MS is less expensive) and results in drug-free remissions for greater than five years in 80 percent of patients. Done right, HSCT is not a cosmetic treatment that temporarily covers disease activity. Both autologous and allogeneic[4]

HSCT can cause the antibody that causes the disease to disappear in most patients.

For the same reasons that I performed the first randomized trial on HSCT for scleroderma and multiple sclerosis, a randomized trial of HSCT for NMO (AQP4 antibody positive) compared to any FDA-approved therapy (there are now three FDA-approved drugs— all expensive, and none eliminate disease-causing AQP4 antibodies) will need to be performed. As in the other randomized trials, patients should be chosen for still having potentially reversible neurologic injury and be allowed to cross over for continued drug failure. The regimen used for HSCT, and patient selection remains the key to a successful outcome.

CHAPTER 7

CHRONIC INFLAMMATORY DEMYELINATING POLYRADICULONEUROPATHY (CIDP): WHAT IS IT?

What is chronic inflammatory demyelinating polyradiculoneuropathy (CIDP)? Even the name is not agreed upon. Because the inflammation includes the nerve root coming out of the spinal cord (in Latin the word *radicular* means *root*), the British call the disease "polyradiculoneuropathy." For some reason, Americans substitute the word polyradiculoneuropathy with the term "polyneuropathy," which means disease involvement (not necessarily even inflammation) of nerves anyplace from the nerve root (that does not have to be involved) to where the nerve adjoins a muscle in the periphery. I will use the British terminology because from my point of view, the British are grammatically correct.

What is CIDP is not just a question readers might ask. It is a question I would ask myself. More appropriately, every time I saw a new patient with CIDP, the first question before entering the room and the last question after examining the patient and leaving the room I would ask myself was, "Is this CIDP?" Trying to figure out an accurate diagnosis for a polyneuropathy or peripheral neuropathy (with or without radicular involvement) can be difficult.

CIDP is an autoimmune neuropathy that involves the peripheral nerves that exit your spinal cord and travel to your muscles. It may occasionally involve the cranial nerves that exit the brain or, rarely, the autonomic nerves that innervate the gut and control blood vessels and heart rate. There are well over one hundred different causes for a peripheral neuropathy. An overwhelming number of peripheral neuropathies are not CIDP but are due to hereditary (genetic), toxic, drug, metabolic, neoplastic (cancer), or infectious causes, or autoimmune diseases that affect multiple organs and are not limited to the peripheral nerves or other neurologic autoimmune diseases that mimic CIDP, such as CANOMAD (which I will not explain because it goes beyond the limits of this book). The point is that many things mimic the clinical symptoms of CIDP, and in my experience, misdiagnosis is common.

CIDP is caused by immune-mediated removal or unwrapping of oligodendrocytes that normally wrap their membrane (myelin) around a peripheral nerve cell. Damage to the neuron (nerve cell) instead of the myelin that envelops the nerve may also be confused with CIDP. I was once referred a patient diagnosed with CIDP for HSCT who, on workup, had a severe degenerative nerve disease called amyotrophic lateral sclerosis (ALS). In North America, ALS is more commonly called Lou Gehrig's disease after the "Iron Horse" New York Yankee power hitter who died two years after his diagnosis. The patient referred to me for "CIDP" was bedridden and could not move her arms or legs. If this had been CIDP, she would have responded to HSCT. (I have treated other bedridden CIDP patients who are now walking without assistance post-treatment.) I told her that she had

ALS (not CIDP) and that a hematopoietic stem cell transplant would not help her. She could not move her arms or hands nor speak—silent tears that screamed despair rolled down her cheeks.

ALS is a neuronal degenerative disease that requires nerve regenerative therapies, which currently do not exist. I felt powerless to help this patient, but this time I did not feel completely lost and without ideas. While I have been treating patients with severe autoimmune diseases with HSCT, I have also been developing a true tissue stem cell regenerative therapy using induced pluripotent stem (IPS) cells (an adult cell genetically reprogrammed to an embryonic stem cell phenotype) to repair damaged nerve cells. Although there are absolutely no guarantees of success, because this type of therapy has worked in animals, I hope, circumstances permitting, to bring it to the bedside.

A patient referred from a prestigious university in the United Kingdom with CIDP for HSCT upon reevaluation had a vitamin deficiency (B12 deficiency). He was sent back to Europe with advice to take a cheap vitamin B12 pill. These cases were not outliers. Of 216 patients referred for HSCT for CIDP, after extensive reevaluation, only sixty-six had CIDP, and of those sixty-six who went through HSCT, three who did not respond to HSCT had another disease that we ourselves also misdiagnosed. After another extensive workup of these three nonresponders, one patient had a genetic (inherited) polyneuropathy and two had a plasma cell dyscrasia (a type of cancer or precancer). I have since written a medical book chapter titled, "Is it CIDP?" where I emphasized that anyone with a diagnosis of treatment-resistant CIDP needs a complete workup for another etiology (or for a no longer autoimmune mediated or "burned out" phase of the disease) before undergoing HSCT and to again repeat the workup for another etiology (cause) for their polyneuropathy if they do not respond to HSCT.

The only drug treatments that have been shown to be beneficial for CIDP are immunoglobulins (intravenous or injected under the skin), plasmapheresis, and steroids. These studies generally enrolled newly diagnosed, treatment-naïve patients and reported one- to two-year outcomes while the patients remained on continuous treatment. We offered HSCT as salvage therapy to patients who were not responding to these treatments. HSCT candidates were often long-term drug treatment failures, and in contrast to drug trials, we reported five-year follow-up with discontinuation of treatments after HSCT. Because of risk benefit concerns, HSCT always has a higher bar to jump.

Down Under

Andrew lived in Australia, and four days after outpatient kidney stone surgery, he felt as exhausted as if he had run a marathon. A few days later, his socks felt like bands pressing on his skin. Removing his shoes and repositioning his socks did not relieve the feeling. A few days later, while playing cricket, his legs felt heavy. One week later, Andrew could not run at all.

His primary care physician did an extensive exam with imaging studies (CT scan, MRI), X-rays, and blood and urine tests. It took a month to get all the tests done and then three months before he could see a neurologist. Andrew told me, "It is not like waiting for Christmas. The wait is mentally paralyzing. You do not know what is wrong, what to expect, or what to do." The neurologist ordered nerve conduction studies (electrophysiology) in Andrew's arms and legs.

After about six months, he got the diagnosis. It was chronic inflammatory demyelinating polyradiculoneuropathy (CIDP). He had never heard of it. This is not unusual. Once when I went to see a CIDP patient in a hospital emergency room, two ER doctors pulled me aside to ask, "What is CIDP?"

Andrew was told that CIDP is treatable. He thought that in a couple of months, he would be back to normal. He was treated with intravenous immunoglobulin (IVIG). The infusion of IVIG was complicated by severe headaches, nausea, and a sense of his head spinning. He tolerated these side effects by putting cold compresses on his head and staying in bed. The IVIG helped by slowing the rate of progressive weakness, numbness, and poor balance, but it did not stop, eliminate, or reverse the disease.

Because his CIDP was worsening despite IVIG, Andrew was started on plasmapheresis. This involved removing the plasma from his blood with a special blood-spinning machine (a centrifuge) and replacing it with salt water, a synthetic plasma, or another person's plasma. Plasmapheresis always left him feeling drained, lightheaded, and faint. Plasmapheresis also failed to arrest or reverse his CIDP. Andrew's doctors tried giving him steroids and a series of different immune drugs individually and in combination. Everything slowed his disease progression, but nothing stopped or reversed it.

Andrew's thinking changed from hoping for normality to worrying what the next stage of disability would do to him. He read and studied everything about CIDP that he could find. He read patient blogs and stories, asked questions on CIDP support group sites, and searched for clinical trials, which he always viewed through the binoculars of skepticism and cynicism, given the gambit of drugs he had already tried. He told me, "It is easy to find an answer; it is finding the right answer that is difficult."

When Andrew learned of a hematopoietic stem cell transplant trial for autoimmune diseases, he wasn't 100 percent sold on the idea and decided that he needed to talk to some other CIDP patients who had been treated with HSCT. He found that a lot of patients were more than happy to share their stories, and that convinced him to try HSCT.

By 2012, twelve years after his diagnosis, Andrew was on an airplane to America for HSCT. Any drug can have multiple rare effects. For Andrew, the cyclophosphamide in the conditioning regimen caused the rare side effect of burning inside the nose, called *wasabi nose*. Fortunately, he responded to antihistamine (Benadryl) and a slower infusion rate.

Andrew did not see any immediate benefits from HSCT, and on the way home to Australia, he wondered if it had even worked. Within the first month at home, his arm pain had disappeared. One and a half months after HSCT, he left a restaurant and realized that he had unintentionally forgotten his walking stick in the restaurant. For the first time in three years, he did not need it. Several months later, Andrew emailed me a video of himself running in a park in Australia. He even returned to playing cricket and scored a few runs. Twelve years earlier, CIDP had forced him to stop playing. This time he decided to retire from cricket on his own terms and with dignity. Since returning to Australia, he has remained off any treatment, and his nerve studies (electrophysiology) have improved. Andrew did not completely return to normal. Some permanent nerve damage remains, but he improved and for the last ten years has required no CIDP medications.

Many years after Andrew's transplant, physicians in Australia invited me to attend a conference and lecture on HSCT for neurological diseases. Andrew came to my talk and was not afraid to interact on an equal level with medical professionals who carry many degrees after their names. Like many of my patients, Andrew knew a lot from his readings and research and his own life experiences with CIDP. He did not just talk the talk. He walked the walk. For me, it felt like seeing a trusted friend in the audience.

Medicine is a jealous profession that demands a lot of time. To compensate for my absence from home, I brought my daughter along with me to Australia for the talk and a detour. We stopped at Hayman Island and then were dropped off on an uninhabited reef. As the boat and outside world vanished over the horizon, her eyes reflected the colors of the underwater corals and beamed with the spirit of adventure. Two giant sea turtles nonchalantly passed close to us, like dogs wanting to be petted. Our hands could have touched them, but it is illegal to touch sea turtles in Australia. The thought had crossed my mind: What if something happened to the outside world and nobody ever returned? As the sun was setting and the tide shifting, the first human souls reappeared as the recovery boat gradually came into sight over the horizon.

Fair

At middle age, Finbarr was living the American dream. He had a great family, a successful career, and was in the best physical condition of his life. His favorite recreational sports were ice hockey, kickboxing, and tennis. In December 2012, after a workout, his nose felt numb and tingly. By February 2013, Finbarr could not feel his feet, and by March he was having trouble walking. In May 2013, the Mayo Clinic diagnosed him with CIDP.

CIDP became a four-year descent into frustration. Steroids did not work, but they did cause weight gain, inability to sleep, and irrational emotions (a common side effect) that were totally foreign to him. IVIG infusions five days every month helped. But at a cost of $20,000 per month, his insurance companies were constantly trying to wean him off the IVIG, after which the CIDP always flared. After restarting IVIG, his recovery was slower and harder than it had previously been. In 2016, when his insurance pulled the plug and stopped approving IVIG, Finbarr's CIDP flared. He became bedridden, unable to walk, had trouble breathing, and was unable to fully move his arms.

After undergoing HSCT in April 2017, Finbarr has remained medication-free, regained his pre-CIDP active lifestyle, and is again playing ice hockey. At a cost for IVIG of $20,000 a month—or $240,000 a year—the transplant that cost $125,000 paid for itself within six months of becoming IVIG-free and, in the last four and a half years, HSCT has saved his insurance company (and society) over one million dollars.

One day out of the blue, Finbarr contacted us and offered to pay for any patient that insurance refused. By coincidence or by fate, another patient was about to start HSCT after fighting and losing his last insurance appeal. The patient's father had raised the money for the hospital by mortgaging his house. We had started the transplant, and the father, having just mortgaged his home to pay the hospital, was sitting in a chair next to his son's bed. When I told him of Finnbarr's offer, he hugged me with a tear running down one cheek. He wanted to know Finbarr's name, but the one and only condition on the money was that his gift remain anonymous. Finbarr did not want to know anything about whom we treated nor vice versa. *Finbarr* is a Celtic name derived from *Fionnbharr*, which means "fair-minded one."

RamG

"RamG" ranked 129th in all of India (a country of over one billion people) on the Indian Institute of Technology Joint Entrance Examination. It is an academic annual examination and the prerequisite for admission to any of the Indian Institutes of Technology. He received a Bachelor of Technology from the Indian Institutes of Technology Madras (IIT-Madras), considered the best institute for higher education in India, and then graduated with a Master of Business Administration (MBA) degree from the Xavier Labour Relations Institute, a private school run by the Society of Jesus (Jesuits) in Jamshedpur. At age thirty-four, while he was working as the chief operating officer in a leading telecom company, the first signs of CIDP—tremors and loss of balance—started.

Over the next nine years, while running the gambit of taking mostly ineffective medications, he continued to decline. By age forty-three, RamG could not button his shirt, could not hold a fork or spoon in his hand, or climb up or down steps without holding on to a railing. He frequently tripped and fell. He was dependent on intravenous immunoglobulin (IVIG). Steroids gave him cataracts that required surgery for both eyes. After nine years of decline, he found through an Internet search that I would be speaking at a medical conference in Bangalore, India. He flew from New Delhi to Bangalore to attend my talk and to introduce himself.

RamG came to America and underwent an uncomplicated transplant. Within six months, he was walking six kilometers a day, buttoning his own shirts, lifting weights, and climbing stairs without any support—all things he had been told that he would never be able to do again. Regaining abilities that he had thought were gone forever awakened within him a desire to become what he had always wanted to be in life. He reinvented his life as a bestselling author, a TEDx speaker, and a much-sought-after keynote speaker. The idea for his first book began while he was in the hospital going through HSCT.

His children were only nine and twelve when he underwent transplant. Now his daughter is a physician in England. His son is pursuing undergraduate studies, majoring in immunology.

After his transplant and after returning to India, RamG arranged for me to speak in New Delhi in order to help initiate a transplant program for neurological diseases that continues to this day. The meeting included a head of neurology from the prestigious All India Institutes of Medical Sciences (AIIMS). When lunchtime came, the Chief of Neurology at AIIMS and I sat next to each other. He was very supportive of HSCT for neurologic diseases. We speculated as to why this approach was not taking off within academia. The answer to this question is not simple and will be discussed in the last chapter of this book.

While in India, RamG took me to a restaurant at a pre-World War II, eighteen-hole British golf club that is still open and still has the elegance and confidence of an optimistic future. RamG is the perfect gentleman—cool under pressure and gracious with success. Like old British royalty himself, he relaxed with a drink and a smile. He told me that his philosophy is never to take himself too seriously but also never accept that something is impossible.

Ben

Ben was an accountant in the United Kingdom who was diagnosed with an unknown (idiopathic) neuropathy in 2001. After two years of testing including a nerve biopsy, he was diagnosed with chronic inflammatory demyelinating polyradiculopathy (CIDP). Despite CIDP, he kept working. By 2007, he was unable to dress himself and relied on others to get around. After seeing him struggle to do the things they took for granted, coworkers in Ben's office would get files for him, bring lunch to his desk, help him put on his jacket or raincoat, and assist him in walking. Ben's mind was sharp, but the nerves running from his spinal cord to his muscles were failing. His ability to do anything was gradually disappearing.

CIDP caused a slow but steady decline in Ben's mobility, strength, and balance. In 2012, he fell and broke his leg, which led to his limited independence evaporating. He always thought he would be there to support his daughters and wife. Instead, he became a burden to them. He underwent multiple types of chronic treatments, including immunoglobulins (IVIG), steroids, and immune drugs such as methotrexate.

Ben's transplant happened in 2013. Instead of the steady decline that had been occurring over the prior twelve years, he experienced a reversal of some neurologic disability, especially during the first two years. For almost a decade since HSCT, Ben has remained off all CIDP medications. His strength and stamina have significantly improved. He can now dress himself, although he still has some problems with buttons due to hand dexterity. Before HSCT, he wore an ankle foot brace (AFO), used a crutch, and needed the support of a companion while walking. He no longer requires a crutch, cane, or companion, but he still wears AFOs due to residual foot drop. Before HSCT he could not lift an empty weight bar off his shoulders. Now he does shoulder presses (military presses) and can lift a bar with 45 kilograms (100 pounds) of weights over his head. Ben started his own accounting company and is now self-employed.

In 2015, two years after HSCT, Ben emailed me saying that for the first time in years, he could jump off the ground. It was not much, but he was able to get off the ground.

Shortly afterward, he sent me a picture of a poster board that had been put together by the school class of his eleven-year-old daughter. The theme was for the kids to write about people they admired. On the poster board there were write-ups and pictures of various famous people including the artist Vincent van Gogh; Nelson Mandela (the father of modern South Africa); Isaac Newton (originator of a mathematical equation for the theory of gravity and inventor of calculus at Cambridge University); Stephen Hawking (theoretical physicist and cosmologist at Cambridge University); and Usain Bolt (the Jamaican sprinter who holds the world record in the 100 and 200 meters). At the center of the poster board was Ben's daughter's contribution, which showed a picture of me and a description of what HSCT had done for her father. Ben's daughters were nine and ten years old at the time of their father's transplant. As of the writing of this book, the eldest daughter is now studying in a British University and the youngest daughter is finishing high school (called Sixth Form in the UK) and will be starting university studies shortly.

The Pilot

Jim was a naval aviator who, after leaving the navy, became a pilot for a major airline. He was in top physical condition when suddenly he lost his balance, could not walk a straight line, could not stand on one foot, and had persistent numbness and pain in his feet and legs. He was diagnosed with CIDP. The Federal Aviation Administration (FAA) abruptly ended his lifelong career as a pilot. Jim made the choice to get HSCT. During the transplant, while Jim was in the hospital, he got influenza and required face mask oxygen, but pulled through just fine.

After the transplant, everything improved. Jim sent me a video of himself standing on one leg with no balance issues. The main residual problem was burning pain in his feet. Burning pain may transiently worsen in a minority of patients with CIDP after HSCT. Nothing seemed to relieve his pain until recommending a nonprescription oral antioxidant called alpha-lipoic acid. His foot pain gradually resolved. Thereafter, CIDP patients were started on oral alpha-lipoic acid during and for several months after transplant, which resulted in only a few of them having subsequent mild cases of foot pain during post-HSCT recovery.

Five years after his transplant, I spoke by phone to Jim's FAA examiner. After our conversation, Jim was approved to return to work as an airline captain and now flies a Boeing flagship 787 on international routes. I enjoy learning the Portuguese language (Brazilian dialect). For me, Latin never became a dead language. Portuguese is living Latin. As I intermittently do some teaching conferences at the University of São Paulo, if our itineraries coincide and Jim flies into São Paulo, I hope to take him to one of my favorite restaurants to try pirarucu (an Indian term meaning red fish), a ten- to fifteen-foot-long torpedolike fish native to the Amazon.

Pirarucu need a natural habitat. Until recently, it was difficult to farm pirarucu in part because they mate for life and if separated will not reproduce. The female pirarucu digs the nest on a shallow bank and, after the eggs hatch, the male pirarucu protects the young from danger by holding them inside his mouth while the female aggressively circles nearby as backup. Except for humans, no carnivore dares to take on two ten-foot-long, four-hundred-pound, torepdo-shaped fish fighting together to protect their young. Their armorlike red scales make them impervious to piranha.

Beach Boy

Dan grew up in California, and his childhood hobbies included skateboarding and surfing. He joined the US Navy at age nineteen and played on the all-Navy soccer team. Each branch of the service has a soccer team selected from the best players in that service. Dan was six feet tall and 185 pounds of muscle. At age twenty-eight, his feet began to tingle and feel numb. He was diagnosed with CIDP and informed by a University of California neurologist that his disease was treatable with intravenous immunoglobulin (IVIG). But the IVIG had no effect. Nothing helped. He also did not respond to plasmapheresis or chemotherapy (Cytoxan).

Six months after the onset of CIDP, he had lost fifty pounds and was in a wheelchair. By the time of transplant, Dan had been out of work for two years, weighed one hundred pounds, could not walk, could not use his hands, and could no longer hold a glass of water. After HSCT, he remained free of all immune drug therapies and his neurologic function slowly returned. By six months post-transplant, he could walk with leg braces, drive a car, and had returned to work as an aerospace engineer. Some permanent nerve damage persisted, as he still could not move his thumbs, toes, or feet.

Dan remained treatment-free for two years. But after two years, he relapsed with sudden onset of clumsiness, tripping, and falling. He restarted IVIG and underwent a second HSCT. This time, after a second HSCT, we continued IVIG on a gradual taper. Dan returned to work within weeks. He remained on IVIG but has tapered to only one infusion every six weeks. It has been four years since the second HSCT. His hands now work well, with the exception of thumbs that have mild deficits (he cannot snap his fingers). He can stand on his tiptoes, but his feet are weak at the ankle (he cannot dorsiflex his foot). He walks using an ankle brace and is again working full time as an aerospace engineer. Because of foot drop, Dan cannot surf standing up. He bodyboards (a short surfboard on which one lies prone) and is back in the ocean bodysurfing.

The Outcome of HSCT on CIDP

What was the outcome of HSCT in sixty CIDP patients who were not going into remission while on standard treatments? People would ask me why I had not published. Like usual, the peer-review process to get the results published was agonizing. Despite drug company publications with one-year follow-up, the one- and two-year outcomes of HSCT were rejected for not long enough follow-up. At five-year submission, one reviewer was then critical for not publishing the results earlier and another rejected the manuscript because the use of an ankle brace (AFO) increased following HSCT. The number of patients requiring assistance to walk with a wheelchair, walker, or cane markedly decreased (Table 6). Only the use of an ankle brace initially increased because as patients became free of wheelchairs, walkers or canes, they were able to use a less-intrusive ankle brace. Over five years after HSCT, on average 80 percent of the patients remained in a treatment-free remission with marked improvements in neurologic function and quality of life.[1] We also published that HSCT is significantly cheaper than continuing IVIG. The average savings over a five-year period were roughly $438,000 US dollars per patient who underwent HSCT.[2]

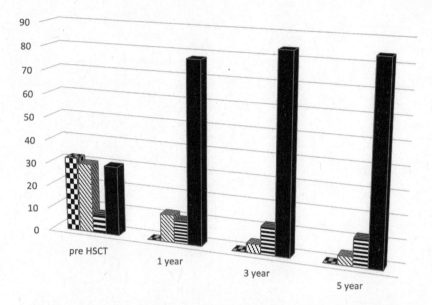

Table 6. CIDP percent ambulatory assistance. Wheelchair walker (checkerboard pattern), cane/crutch (lines sloping down at 45 degrees), ankle brace (AFO) (horizontal lines), no assistance (solid column) pre-HSCT and 1, 3, and 5 years post-HSCT

In 2020 we published the results of the first prospective trial of HSCT for CIDP. A randomized trial for final proof will be needed. As always, results will depend on the conditioning regimen and patient selection; that is, making sure that the patient actually has CIDP and that it is still active (not burned out, nonactive disease with permanent neuronal degeneration).

CHAPTER 8

CROHN'S DISEASE: SHELL SHOCK

As a young assistant professor who was not even a gastroenterologist, I approached the Professor and Chief of Gastroenterology, Dr. Craig about the concept of HSCT for Crohn's disease. His area of expertise is Crohn's disease, and he liked the idea. He was, for me and for the project, a godsend to work with. When we admitted a Crohn's patient for HSCT, Dr. Craig would write under his patient note: "Go, stem cells." After Dr. Craig retired, he sent me a lay book that he had published. In it he included a handwritten inscription that said, "My involvement in your program was one of the smartest things that I did." Dr. Craig remains a valued, respected friend to this day.

Like multiple sclerosis, Crohn's disease does not in general decrease life expectancy, but it can make life feel like it's not worth living. In adult onset, it will frequently demolish a marriage. In childhood onset, it is a thief that robs a person of adolescence. The chronic pain and psychological effects of losing control of the bowels causes severe psychological stress especially during the teenage years, but psychological damage can occur regardless of the age of onset.

While Crohn's disease primarily affects the gut (gastrointestinal tract), it is an immune-mediated disease and, like the immune system itself, has far-reaching effects that may occur outside of the primary organ system involved. Other organs that can be affected by Crohn's are the joints, skin, eyes, liver (bile tract), and lungs.

I once had a Crohn's patient referred from Baylor College of Medicine in Houston, where I had been the Chief Medical Resident. As Chief Resident, I ran the morning report and taught other residents. The Chair of Medicine, Dr. Lynch, was the most knowledgeable clinician I have ever known. It was always a little intimidating to present in front of him. He was not mean or rude in any way. He just seemed to know everything about every medical disease.

Decades later, Baylor referred a Crohn's patient to me for HSCT. On workup, nodules or lesions (granulomas) were found in the patient's lungs. Dr. Lynch was involved in the care of this patient and inquired over the telephone about the cause of these lung nodules (granulomas). As I explained the Crohn's-related immune etiology, I felt that day the hallmark of a maestro teacher—pride in his pupil.

Crohn's involvement of the gut may be luminal (on the interior surface), stricturing (closing shut the bowel with obstruction), or fistulizing (penetrating through the bowel to make an opening or a new tract that exits outside the body or sometimes to another part of the bowel or another organ, such as the bladder) (Figure 4).

Long before I had the idea of perfecting HSCT for Crohn's disease, a patient complained that when he would try to urinate, foul air blew out of his phallus (male organ). He had Crohn's disease that had drilled a tract (fistula) from his bowel into his bladder. Flatulence (bowel gas) would blow out when trying to urinate.

Fistulae can also make new bowel tracts to the vagina and to the abdominal wall. In one case, I saw a patient where the fistula tracked down the inside of her thigh and exited with stool dripping out just above her knee. Because fistulae lack a natural anatomical

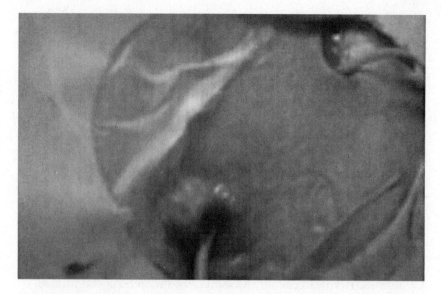

Figure 4 - Crohn fistulae. Lower left is anal opening. Top right is site of fistula exiting the skin. A rubber thread is passed from the rectum/anus through the fistula to its exit to demonstrate continuity. The picture is not from a patient mentioned herein.

anal muscle, stool leaks out of the end of the fistula into the vagina, or onto the abdomen, thigh, or wherever the fistula exits the body. The psychological consequences of stool dripping out of these locations are devastating.

In general, drug trials for FDA approval for new Crohn's treatments do not include patients with stricturing, penetrating, or fistulizing disease (only luminal); do not report more than one or two years of follow-up; do not enroll previously treated patients; do not in general report quality of life or costs; and allow for simultaneous treatment with other drugs. The drug is administered chronically without expecting it to be discontinued. Typically, a Crohn's drug study will allow and is not altered by use of other drugs or surgery while on the experimental drug. (Some trials report duration of being steroid-free, but other drugs and surgery are allowed.)

In contrast, for HSCT we selected heavily pretreated patients with disease that had failed the currently approved drugs at that time and, besides severe luminal disease, had penetrating, stricturing, and/or fistulizing disease. We treated just once and then discharged them with no drugs and reported five-year follow-ups with patients off all immune medications.

Our initial trial used an autologous stem cell-selected graft with a nonmyeloablative regimen of cyclophosphamide and ATG. The one-year results were very encouraging, but by three years, 50 percent relapsed, and by five years, 80 percent relapsed.[1] A few remained in longer-term remission, but most had relapsed by five years. The gastro-enterologist was not discouraged because, despite relapse, these patients' Crohn's activity was generally less severe and more easily controlled.

I have a surgeon's mentality and desire a one-time intervention. I wanted to convert chronic autoimmune diseases into a one-time reversible illness. Thus, I designed a new approach for Crohn's disease.

I elected not to use autologous stem cells but instead to infuse allo-geneic stem cells—that is, stem cells mostly sourced from another person's immunologically matched umbilical cord blood. Another person's umbilical cord blood does not contain any potentially contaminating Crohn's disease-causing immune cells and may provide an additional allogeneic (foreign cell) disease-ameliorating effect. The danger is that the umbilical cord blood cells may not take to the patient and will either disappear entirely or alternatively attack the patient and cause another autoimmune disease called graft-versus-host disease (GVHD).

The protocol was designed to prevent GVHD and to allow recon-stitution of autologous blood cells if the allogeneic umbilical cord blood did not persist (engraft). This was fortuitous as the umbilical cord cells did not persist. Dose escalation of the conditioning regi-men to try to ensure umbilical cord blood survival was complicated at maximal dose by one patient's death. When that happened, I volun-tarily stopped study enrollment and continued to follow the already transplanted patients. We reported that at five years follow-up, all the patients remained off immune medications and had no Crohn's disease noted by clinical symptoms, external imaging scans, or internal imaging with colonoscopy, no histologic disease on random colonic biopsy, and the damaged areas of the gut had healed.[2]

The details of why allogeneic umbilical cord blood worked go beyond the scope of this book. In honesty, I am not 100 percent sure why. The cells did not persist (engraft). Autologous (self) cells reconstituted the immune system. Future studies are needed, but because the umbilical cord blood worked without the cells engrafting in the patient, I suspect the results were from the conditioning regimen—Cytoxan, fludarabine (both immune-specific chemotherapy drugs); alemtuzumab (an antibody to immune cells); and six months of tacrolimus (an oral immune suppressant), and the fact that the umbilical cord contained no disease reactivating immune cells (lymphocytes) that may be present within an infused autologous graft. It was important to note for future studies that it worked even at the lowest and safer conditioning regimen dosing. What needs to be repeatedly emphasized is that results and toxicity of HSCT for each autoimmune disease depend on the conditioning regimen and on patient selection for that disease.

As I followed these transplanted patients, I saw for the first time in a Crohn's disease treatment that HSCT, a one-time treatment, resulted in long-term, ten- to twelve-year treatment-free disease remissions without imaging, endoscopic or microscopic (histologic) evidence of disease, and it did this in patients with severe refractory disease. These patients are the primer needed for further studies, and herein are some of their stories.

Partial Colectomy Failed

Patrick was diagnosed with Crohn's disease in 2006 when he was sixteen years old. At first, his disease was well controlled with medications. While in college, his Crohn's became more aggressive with unpredictable diarrhea and abdominal pains. On average, one to three times per year he was hospitalized for severe abdominal pain and/or bowel obstruction. He had tried the gambit of available immune medications (azathioprine, methotrexate, mercaptopurine, Humira, Remicade, Tysabri, and steroids).

His Crohn's caused perianal abscesses and nonhealing perianal fistulae. About two-thirds of his colon (large bowel) was so severely damaged that it was surgically removed (partial colectomy). The disease flared in the remaining colon that was left inside his body.

Because nothing was stopping his disease, Patrick went to two different Mayo Clinic centers and to Harvard's Massachusetts General Hospital in Boston for second and third opinions. The verdict was unanimous: he was told that he needed surgery to removing his entire colon (a total colectomy). The problem was that after a total colectomy, Patrick would have a bag (colostomy bag) that hung outside of his belly continuously collecting stool (feces).

Nobody, especially no young, single person, wants a colostomy bag. It is an intimacy buzzkill. The second problem is that Crohn's disease may reoccur any place along the digestive tract, from the mouth to the anus. Removing the entire colon (large bowel) does not remove the risk for uncontrolled Crohn's disease in the small bowel. Finally, once surgically removed, you cannot get your colon back. It is gone forever. Standard of care colectomy is accepted as state of the art by physicians, but it is a barbaric, primitive, brutal, and psychologically traumatic event for most patients.

Patrick refused a total colectomy. His mother turned to her own research and found out about HSCT on the Internet. Patrick underwent HSCT in 2014 at the age of twenty-six after eight years of suffering from Crohn's disease. His symptoms disappeared the day he left the hospital. He has had no medications and no symptoms for the last eight years since transplant. He works full time as an engineer, has normal bowel control and bowel habits, and is an aquarist who is especially good with exotic coral reefs.

At the time of this writing, he is engaged to be married. His own gastroenterologist had never heard about HSCT for Crohn's disease, and Patrick has had no need to go back. For his gastroenterologist's own knowledge, I wish Patrick had returned. But I understand. As another patient wisely once told me, "It is sometimes better to leave the past in the past."

Straight-A Student and Athlete

Anthony was diagnosed with an indeterminate colitis at age fifteen. His symptoms started abruptly one Thanksgiving with diarrhea, nausea, vomiting, and rectal bleeding. A digital camera was inserted via the anus to inspect the inside of his colon, and it revealed pan colitis (inflammation of the entire colon). Total parenteral nutrition (TPN), with feeding intravenously and taking nothing by mouth, did not relieve his symptoms. The drugs mesalamine (Pentasa), steroids, and Remicade were started, but they did not work either. Anthony lost twenty-six pounds. Remicade had to be stopped due to drug-induced, life-threatening collapse of his airway called anaphylaxis, where his neck and tongue swelled, making breathing difficult.

For six months, Anthony was in and out of Children's Hospital of Philadelphia. On his sixteenth birthday he was started on the drug Humira, after which he felt good for about two weeks before it stopped working. He had developed antibodies to Humira. Despite not being approved for pediatric use, Children's Hospital of Philadelphia got permission to start Anthony on another drug, Cimzia (certolizumab). He remained on Cimzia, steroids, and methotrexate. The steroids caused severe cystic acne on his face, chest, and back.

A rectal abscess, a painful pocket of pus, developed. After surgery to drain the abscess and a second colonoscopy, Anthony was diagnosed with Crohn's disease. He received a seton, which is a cotton plug surgically placed in the abscess and left sticking out of his skin. It helps the abscess to drain or decompress, but it is not a cure.

Before Crohn's, Anthony had been a straight A student and a three-sport athlete. He was slated for a D-1 (Division 1) college baseball career. After Crohn's, Anthony had to be homeschooled and missed two years of high school. Shortly after starting college, he was again hospitalized and started on tube feedings (a tube was put through his nose and into his stomach to provide nutrition) to help him gain weight.

When Anthony was nineteen, surgical removal of the entire large bowel (total colectomy) was recommended. In order to rest his colon and to buy time to find and get a hematopoietic stem cell transplant, he instead underwent a diverting ileostomy. In other words, his small bowel was surgically cut off from his colon and reconnected to a surgical opening made in the skin of the belly to allow feces to drip into a bag kept on his belly.

The diverting ileostomy prolapsed, in other words his small intestine spilled outside of his abdomen. Attempts to surgically close the wound failed. It was left to heal by secondary intention—that is, the wound was left open to air to heal by itself. Anthony had to lie on his back for five weeks. He could not turn to either side. His abdomen was flayed open like a fish that had been gutted. He emotionally crashed. Crohn's had killed his spirit, along with his once-admirable sense of humor. He became absent in mind and spirit and secluded himself in solitude. He was diagnosed with post-traumatic stress disorder (PTSD) and major depressive disorder.

Chronic nausea and weight loss remained a problem. The only medication that helped his nausea and boosted his appetite, despite not being able to eat anything but a bland diet, was marijuana, which he found himself needing to use chronically.

Anthony's transplant took place in 2014. The Crohn's abated almost immediately, but the first year after HSCT was rough with a

CROHN'S DISEASE: SHELL SHOCK

lot of ups and downs. Since then, it has been smooth sailing. Anthony has been off all medications for eight years with no symptoms or evidence of Crohn's disease and no nausea. He eats what he wants, returned to college, and graduated with a double major in radio and television and film sports communication and a minor in journalism. He works full time, lives with two buddies, and has a girlfriend. He no longer uses marijuana and is living a full life, traveling when he can and looking forward to the future.

Fighting the Humiliation of Crohn's

At age ten, Krista developed symptoms of abdominal pain, constipation, and bloody stools and was diagnosed with Crohn's disease at age twelve. She ate very little, and her growth was retarded. Her height and weight were in the third percentile of what a normal twelve-year-old girl should be. After her first colonoscopy, she was started on steroids (prednisone) and mercaptopurine. A few months later, she had to be hospitalized and put on bowel rest with nothing taken by mouth for five continuous months in a treatment called total parenteral nutrition (TPN). All calories (protein, fats, minerals, and vitamins) and fluids were infused intravenously into her veins. Steroids helped, and she remained on them every day until age fourteen, when they were stopped due to steroid-induced osteoporosis (weak, brittle bones) that normally is a problem with older, geriatric-age patients. Two years of taking steroids as a child had caused Krista's bones to become weak and her growth plates to stop growing. Different monoclonal antibodies (adalimumab, infliximab, certolizumab) used to treat Crohn's were tried, but none worked for her.

Repeat bowel rest and TPN became ineffective and no longer abated Krista's symptoms. A Crohn's-related perianal abscess developed, and different antibiotics were tried. The most effective for her was the tuberculosis drug rifampin, but it caused persistent nausea and had to be stopped after six months.

By age seventeen she had begun a downward spiral. Once she went to a prom dance, but it was a disaster. Her mom had to come pick her up because of Krista's severe abdominal cramps, pain, and diarrhea. Throughout her teenage years, she was confined to bed all day and did not date or go out. She confided, "When you are a teenager and are in and out of the hospital all the time and sick with uncontrollable pain and diarrhea, you have no self-confidence, no self-esteem." As a teenage girl, she was embarrassed to tell anyone about her condition. Nobody in her school knew, except her best friend, who kept her secret. Her teachers knew and respected her by also keeping her secret. Crohn's had exiled her. It made her feel shame for what it was doing to her. She was relentlessly victimized by a heartless, unreasoning, invisible assailant that made her ashamed for the domestic violence it was committing upon her body.

A drug used to prevent organ transplant rejection (tacrolimus) was started but was only marginally effective. Krista weighed 85 pounds and could not stand up without severe abdominal pain. Her physicians wanted to remove her entire colon and have her live with a stool collection bag. Krista felt like this was the last straw. Hopelessness had boxed her into a corner of isolation, despair, and defeat.

Krista's brother did not accept the medical experts' opinion to get a total colectomy. He knew what that would do to what was left of his sister. He googled everything he could find on Crohn's disease and found out about HSCT. In 2011, at the age of twenty, Krista underwent HSCT.

It has now been eleven years after transplant. Since HSCT, she has been on no medications and has had no bowel symptoms. Her weight became normal for the first time in her life. She went to college, became a registered nurse, got a job in a medical surgical unit, fell in love, got married, and is now the mother of two children. She suffered from Crohn's from age ten until she was twenty years old and could only dream of a normal life. Now Krista lives a normal, full life. She is a wife, a mother, a nurse, and she loves cooking and being outdoors.

Ten years after HSCT, Krista sent me an email. It read, "I wanted to say thank you so much for what you do, I honestly don't know where I would be without having had this transplant."

Evolution

Patrick (a different Patrick than in one of the previous stories) was ten years old when he developed Crohn's with diarrhea and stomach cramps. After a tube with a camera on it was placed down his mouth and up his rectum and colon, he was diagnosed and started on prednisone and other drugs. He was dependent on prednisone, often taking it at high doses. His doctors would add other drugs in an attempt to decrease the amount of prednisone, but his symptoms would flare up. The long-term effects of chronic prednisone or any chronic steroid are legion. The drug can destroy bones and growth plates, so after three years his doctors switched Patrick from prednisone to a form of steroid called Entocort (Budesonide) that coats the inside of the gut with less systemic absorption into the blood.

Patrick tried a variety of monoclonal antibodies: infliximab (Remicade) for two years, adalimumab (Humira) for two to three years, then Certolizumab (Cimzia) for several more years. Each partially worked at first but then gradually became ineffective. He continued to have bloody diarrhea, joint pains, fatigue, and sores in his mouth.

Patrick lost his childhood and teenage years to Crohn's. He had to be homeschooled from fourth through twelfth grades. Abdominal pain was fairly constant. Quick access to a bathroom was essential. He could not continue playing sports and had no dating life. As Patrick said to me, "Crohn's is not very sexy." His rational mind knew that his existence was a lifetime of suffering, but his soul kept the possibility alive that he might someday, somehow, be healthy. Crohn's had stripped him of any sense of normalcy, but he would still dream about becoming healthy and being able to live a full life where he could be free of symptoms and pain.

At age twenty, after ten years of suffering from Crohn's disease, Patrick underwent HSCT. The transplant was uncomplicated. For the first six months after HSCT, he had some common ups and downs, but by nine months he was symptom- and drug-free. Before HSCT, Patrick's workup had revealed a large bowel stricture that threatened to cause total obstruction in the future. He was informed that he might still need surgery after transplant. But without any other treatment, the large bowel stricture completely disappeared on its own after transplantation. I have seen this in other patients as well, where large bowel (but not small bowel) colonic strictures completely resolved after HSCT. This also occurs with fistula. They gradually heal after HSCT. Post-transplant, Patrick has remained drug-free and disease-free and has been on no medications for eleven years.

Patrick finished college. He studied (in part) abroad in Sweden at Uppsala University. I still find that life is full of the extraordinary. I have spoken on several occasions at Uppsala University. I have walked around that campus a number of times, and Uppsala University was one of the centers for my randomized HSCT trial for MS. We did not bump into each other (universities are big places), but Patrick and I were undoubtedly there at the same time.

The recovery from a medical disease was only part of Patrick's evolution. After his Crohn's disease went into remission, he suffered, like so many of my patients, from post-traumatic stress disorder (PTSD), which is a syndrome first described in World War I soldiers after prolonged combat exposure. The original name used for PTSD was "shell shock." Like Charlie of the short story and play *Flowers for Algernon*, when you recover and are free from a chronic disease, the spirit and soul must still recover. Patrick has his own profound and severe PTSD journey that he will tell in his own way, on his own time. He recovered through many methods, including dance, learning to relate with his perceptions and sensory world, meditation, and profoundly supportive relationships. I titled this section "Evolution" because recovery from a chronic disease is both a physical and spiritual evolution and because Patrick's website is about evolution, where he wrote in a poem:

"Only you can do you
So do it
Only you can be you
So be it."

CHAPTER 9

WHY CAN'T I GET HSCT?: EYES WIDE CLOSED

Patients have asked me why people and institutions are not shouting from the rooftops about hematopoietic stem cell transplantation for autoimmune diseases. Some want to know why they personally cannot get or have not heard about HSCT.

The problems mentioned herein are only a few of many stories. As in all walks of life, jealousy, politics, and hidden agendas all play a role. But there is no intentional malevolence on the part of most people. Rather, the failure to recognize, accept, or offer HSCT arises from systemic, subtle, and indirect but ingrained patterns within the larger medical field that have contributed to long-established and reinforced patterns of thinking and acting.

These Entities Are *Not* Responsible for Hindering HSCT

Food and Drug Administration (FDA)

Patients often direct their frustration toward the FDA. They want to know why the FDA has not approved this procedure. I understand my patients' vexation, but the FDA is not directly the issue and is not to blame.

The FDA controls the licensing, approval, and safety of new drugs. A patient's hematopoietic (blood) stem cells, when used for HSCT, are not a drug. Hematopoietic stem cells are not manufactured or patented and cannot be licensed for the exclusive profit of some company, person, or entity. In my protocols, the hematopoietic stem cells are not manipulated or modified (beyond freezing/storage) and are being used for a homologous rather than a heterologous purpose. A homologous purpose means that the hematopoietic stem cell is being used for its normal physiologic function.[1]

An analogy of a homologous purpose is a red blood cell transfusion that is infused into a patient's vein. If a patient is losing blood (from a traumatic accident for example), red blood cells are infused to stabilize the patient. These red blood cells are collected without compensation from volunteers. No company owns or has an FDA license to monopolize the sale of red blood cells.

Since most hematopoietic stem cell transplants for autoimmune diseases are autologous—that is, the cells were collected from the patient themselves—a better analogy is a surgeon who collects a unit of red blood cells from a patient well before an elective surgery and then reinfuses the patient's own red blood cells post-operatively (after surgery) to hasten recovery from the operation. No company manufactures, owns, or has a license on a patient's own red blood cells. No investigational new drug (IND) number would be licensed by the FDA.

Hematopoietic stem cells, when used for autoimmune disease, are also a transfusion blood product, not a therapeutic investigational new drug (IND). Falling under FDA licensing would be nonsensical because nobody made your own blood or blood (hematopoietic) stem cells. It would also be unethical. If a government could license your own blood products, who would be authorized to claim it: a drug company, a person, an entity, an organization, a committee, or the government itself? If something or someone other than you could own and license your blood, then they could own your finger, your arm, your leg, or any of your organs. We have already witnessed the historical horror of owning another person or parts of that person. It is called "slavery."

What about the drugs infused in the conditioning regimen? Once a drug is approved and licensed by the FDA, all physicians have the right to use the drug for off-label indications, provided it is administered within published acceptable dosages, and no one is trying to gain a license for that indication. In fact, the drugs used for HSCT conditioning regimens have had their patents expire long ago, which means that no company would invest in the drug because, without patent protection, a company cannot monopolize or profit from that drug and cannot recover their expenses from developing the drug or from doing the clinical studies. Anybody can make and sell it as a generic drug. Once a patent expires, the cost (and profit) of a drug markedly falls.

In clinical practice, many drugs are used off-label all the time. This is one reason why physicians are trained for literally more than a decade before obtaining a license to prescribe medicines. Their medical degree (MD) and state or government license give them that right. If physicians were not licensed to do this, patients would suffer and die virtually all the time. For example, steroids and Cytoxan are used for almost every autoimmune disease, including all the diseases discussed in this book, yet neither steroids nor Cytoxan have ever been FDA-approved for these indications, nor will they be. The patents have expired.

The drugs used in conditioning regimens for HSCT of patients with leukemia and cancers have never been FDA-approved for those indications, but transplants for cancer using transplant dosing of chemotherapy and other drugs (e.g., biologics) have been ongoing since the 1960s. The doses of drugs used in autoimmune transplant regimens have already been used and published for lymphoma, leukemia, and for hematologic autoimmune diseases such as aplastic anemia, for which transplant doses of cyclophosphamide and anti-thymocyte globulin (ATG) have been used since the 1960s.

Knowing all this, I idealistically and voluntarily submitted my protocols to the FDA. This left me open to an onsite FDA visit. The way the FDA operates is that, rather than documenting the good, the FDA documents only errors including administrative errors. The FDA does so in the minutia of the smallest of details, which ended up interrupting eight months of my life. What is not stated is that I did not need to go through the FDA. It was voluntary, and the published outcome data was entirely accurate. The FDA recommended no changes in my protocols and no changes in drugs or dosing or in patient eligibility. But, as mentioned, they do not comment on the positive.

Aleksandr Solzhenitsyn, author of *The Cancer Ward*, wrote: "It was wrong to be too pragmatic, to judge people solely by results; it was more humane to judge by intentions."[2] To which it may be added and for which anyone caught in a bureaucratic vortex can attest: Bureaucracy judges neither by intentions nor results but by paperwork.

I have always known that to ensure accuracy, you go to the source. After the site visit completion and after all eight months of paperwork, I went to the source. I requested, and the FDA was kind enough to allow me, to meet with the Director of the Office of Cell and Gene Therapy in the FDA Maryland White Oak Campus. (The new FDA commissioner could not attend due to briefings for Senate confirmation.) After the meeting, the director apologized on behalf of the FDA and confirmed that I had never needed to submit protocols to the FDA.

Nevertheless, the FDA does not publish apologies online, nor would I expect such an agency to do that. I doubt that anyone within the FDA would want to accept the responsibility to do that. I was just thankful that the director agreed to a meeting and confirmed my understandings of regulations. But it is amazing the degree of confusion that can be sown on social media or by unvetted and unregulated bloggers, who can sometimes push misinformation into the mainstream media.

Pharmaceutical (Drug) Companies

Patients have frequently expressed frustration toward pharmaceutical companies for possible hindrance in developing HSCT for autoimmune diseases. But drug companies are not directly the problem. Drug companies have no interest in HSCT because there is no return on investment for them. But neither did any drug company ever do anything to belittle or hinder HSCT. Doing so would not serve their financial interests.

Once, while traveling on United Airlines, a purser told me that an entire floor of the Willis Tower, a 108-story skyscraper in Chicago, is devoted to monitoring social media comments made by United passengers in order to rapidly defuse negative remarks. In terms of public relations, to which big pharmaceutical companies are very attentive, belittling HSCT or belittling physicians would be suicidal. For drug companies, HSCT does not benefit them but neither does it threaten them. It is a nonentity to them. They do not help, nor do they hinder, its development.

Insurance Companies

Insurance, depending on the company (as described in the MS chapter), can definitely be an issue for patients seeking HSCT, and a rare medical director can be incalcitrant. But in truth, most private insurance companies cover HSCT. Approval may require months, sometimes longer than six to ten months, and multiple appeals, but in the end, most medical insurance companies eventually pay.

Medicine is complex and highly subspecialized, and it is impossible for anyone or any insurance company to stay truly informed and up-to-date on all treatments or on all aspects of an individual patient's circumstances. The key is being able to speak directly with a person or committee making the decision and to get them the information. Part of the rationale for my recent medical textbook (Burt et al., *Hematopoietic Stem Cell Transplantation and Cellular Therapies for Autoimmune Diseases*, CRC Press, 2021), this lay book, a website (www.astemcelljourney.com), and numerous medical journal publications is to help disseminate accurate information to medical professionals, medical insurers, and patients.

Insurance companies, governing committees, and governments establish broad policies. The problem that exists in all organizations is a breakdown in what is best for a particular individual versus implementation of a concept for the "greater good." The bigger the organization (or government), the more an individual and their circumstances are lost in the banality of administrative regulations.

Conflicts arise between prioritizing the individual versus designing general policies for society. Different people put different weights on each side of that scale. Society and policies provide a framework to prevent people from running amok. On the other hand, crushing an individual undermines the core pillars that constitute a society. As the Zimbabwean-born philosopher Matshona Dhliwayo said, "Better an individual and you better society." Or as the Indian mystic Rajneesh, whose beliefs contributed to Western New Age thinking, said, "To me each individual is far more valuable than society as a whole." For me as a physician, my responsibility is to always do the best for the individual patient in front of me. If I did otherwise, then trust between patient and physician would be lost and, without trust, all future actions become suspect.

The Real Obstacles to HSCT

The real hindrances to developing HSCT for autoimmune diseases are more oblique, but in combination they have a significant impact on restraining this field.

Risk Benefit

Is the risk of HSCT worth the benefit? Physicians are risk-averse. There is a medical axiom, "Do no harm." Hospitals are complex, and patient dynamics may change rapidly, which is an environment for errors to multiply and for patients to get hurt. In addition, all drugs and all operations have both short-term and long-term complications. For some reason, young doctors think of drugs as miracle pills, and they can be, but all drugs have toxicities. When a patient is having a medical problem, the first thing a physician should do is examine the medications they are taking. Iatrogenic causes, for example physician-prescribed medications, are not infrequently the culprit. And HSCT, due to the high dose of drugs in the conditioning regimen, can have serious adverse consequences. No patient can be promised a good outcome. It is for this reason that I have argued for the less toxic nonmyeloablative conditioning regimens instead of myeloablative conditioning regimens that were originally designed for cancers.

Given that all treatments and all prescription drugs are double-edged swords (even a bag of normal saline [salt water] can be lethal for a patient with scleroderma, Figure 3), how does one ethically treat anyone? The key is informed consent. All patients need to be informed of not just possible benefits but of all risks, including differences between nonmyeloablative and myeloablative regimens and the potential for unknown complications. Ethically, it is or should ultimately be the patient's decision, not the government's nor the insurance companies' decisions.

When I first floated the concept of HSCT for autoimmune diseases, many medical specialists thought it was too risky an idea. In an unanticipated reversal of roles, I became the one arguing that aggressive myeloablative conditioning regimens (Tables 4 and 5) are too toxic, too potentially risky, and not necessary for autoimmune diseases.

When any treatment is offered, you want to make it as safe as possible. For that reason, I have relentlessly advocated for safer, non-myeloablative regimens. As I have said throughout this book, toxicity and outcome depend on the regimen (and patient selection). If you do not know which regimen is more effective, then start with the safest conditioning regimen.

At some point, when increasing the intensity of conditioning regimens, the toxicity will outweigh the benefit. Maximally aggressive regimens are not known to be superior in outcome. In general, the more aggressive the regimen, the more toxic and expensive it becomes. Finding the right HSCT conditioning regimen is like trying to find a planet in the "Goldilocks Zone" that supports life—not too hot, not too cold—that is not too intense, not too weak. The default in the American medical system seems to favor the most aggressive and most expensive.

Homeless

Each organ system has a board-certified subspecialty such as cardiology (the heart); nephrology (the kidneys); dermatology (the skin); ophthalmology (the eyes); pulmonology (the lungs); neurology (the brain and nervous system); rheumatology (traditionally, joints, muscles, and ligaments); otolaryngology (the ears, eyes, and throat); obstetrics and gynecology (pregnancy, birth, and female organs); urology (the urinary tract); hematology (diseases of the blood); and psychiatry (mental and emotional disorders).

Certain procedures or aspects of medical care have also been organized into their own training programs and board certifications, such as radiology (X-rays and imaging), medical intensive care, and emergency medicine (emergency room physicians). Some diseases are also organized into their own subspecialty training programs and board examinations, for example, oncology (cancer).

As a scholastic discipline, autoimmune diseases do not have a home. I was originally trained in the field of hematology and then subspecialized in HSCT for leukemia before proposing the idea of HSCT for autoimmune diseases. I had to train myself in each new autoimmune disease.

Autoimmune diseases do not have a defined department. There are more than seventy-five different autoimmune diseases (Figure 5) that are clinically separated into numerous different medical departments or divisions. For example, Crohn's disease is within gastroenterology, systemic sclerosis is in rheumatology (and pulmonary, renal, and cardiology), and multiple sclerosis is a part of neurology.

When medicine was first organized into subspecialties, diseases were categorized and organized by organ systems that could be visualized. Physicians had no knowledge of and did not have microscopes to visualize immune cells that circulate pretty much everywhere throughout the body. Once immune cells were discovered to be the cause of autoimmune diseases, immunology departments arose to specialize in the basic research of immune cells. But the diverse clinical presentation of different autoimmune diseases had already been assigned to numerous different organ-specific medical departments or divisions. The result of this structure is that autoimmune disease specialists do not know, perform, or understand hematopoietic stem cell transplantation and are reluctant to refer patients, while hematopoietic stem cell transplant specialists do not know or understand autoimmune diseases.

AFFECTED BODY PART	DISORDER	FREQUENCY IN POPULATION (Approx ratio of people living with the diagnosis)
NEUROLOGY — NERVE & BRAIN	Multiple sclerosis	1 in 1,000
	Narcolepsy	1 in 10,000
	Myasthenia gravis	1 in 10,000
	Chronic inflammatory demyelinating polyneuropathy	1 in 100,000
	Guillain-Barré syndrome	1 in 100,000
	Hashimoto's encephalopathy	1 in 100,000
	Neuromyelitis optica	1 in 100,000
	Acute disseminated encephalomyelitis	1 in a million
	PANDAS	< 1 in a million
	Miller Fisher syndrome	< 1 in a million
	Autoimmune inner ear disease	< 1 in a million
	Vogt-Koyanagi-Harada syndrome	< 1 in a million
	Morvan's syndrome	< 1 in a million
	Stiff-person syndrome	< 1 in a million
	Isaac's syndrome/acquired neuromyotonia	< 1 in a million
	Rasmussen's encephalitis	< 1 in a million
DERMATOLOGY — SKIN & MUCOUS MEMBRANE	Psoriasis	More than 1 in 100
	Vitiligo	1 in 1,000
	Alopecia areata	1 in 1,000
	Dermatitis herpetiformis	1 in 10,000
	Discoid lupus erythematosus	1 in 10,000
	Bullous pemphigoid	1 in 100,000
	Linear morphea	1 in 100,000
	Pemphigus foliaceus	1 in 100,000
	Epidermolysis bullosa acquisita	1 in a million
	Phemphigus foliaceus	1 in a million
	Cicatricial pemphigoid	1 in a million
ENDOCRINOLOGY — ENDOCRINE SYSTEM	Hashimoto's autoimmune thyroiditis	1 in 100
	Graves' disease	1 in 100
	Type 1 diabetes mellitus	1 in 1,000
	Addison's disease	1 in 10,000
	Autoimmune polyglandular syndrome 2	1 in 100,000
	Autoimmune polyglandular syndrome 1	1 in 100,000
	Autoimmune orchitis	< 1 in a million
	IPEX syndrome	< 1 in a million
	Autoimmune hypoparathyroidism	< 1 in a million
	Autoimmune polyglandular syndrome 3	< 1 in a million
	Autoimmune hypophysitis	< 1 in a million
	Autoimmune oophoritis	< 1 in a million
GASTROENTEROLOGY — DIGESTIVE SYSTEMS	Celiac disease	1 in 100
	Pernicious anemia	1 in 100
	Ulcerative colitis	1 in 1,000
	Crohn's disease	1 in 10,000
	Type 1 autoimmune hepatitis	1 in 100,000
	Primary sclerosing cholangitis	< 1 in a million
	Type 2 autoimmune hepatitis	< 1 in a million
	Autoimmune pancreatitis	< 1 in a million

AFFECTED BODY PART	DISORDER	FREQUENCY IN POPULATION (Approx ratio of people living with the diagnosis)
RHEUMATOLOGY — MUSCLE & BONES	Rheumatoid arthritis	1 in 100
	Polymyositis/dermatomyositis	1 in 10,000
	Still's disease	1 in 100,000
	Relapsing Polychrondritis	1 in a million
RHEUMATOLOGY — BLOOD VESSELS	Rheumatic fever	1 in 1,000
	Temporal arteritis	1 in 10,000
	Kawasaki disease	1 in 10,000
	Polyarteritis nodosa	1 in 10,000
	Granulomatosis with polyangiitis	1 in 100,000
	Microscopic polyangiitis	1 in 100,000
	Takayasu arteritis	1 in a million
RHEUMATOLOGY — MULTIPLE ORGANS	Systemic lupus erythematosus	1 in 10,000
	Systemic sclerosis	1 in 10,000
	Sjögren's syndrome	1 in 10,000
	CREST syndrome	1 in 10,000
	Mixed connective tissue disease	1 in 100,000
	Eosinophilic granulomatosis with polyangiitis	1 in a million
HEMATOLOGY — BLOOD & BONE MARROW	Immune thrombocytopenic purpura	1 in 1,000
	Antiphospholipid syndrome	1 in 10,000
	Felty's syndrome	1 in 100,000
	Autoimmune hemolytic anemia	1 in 100,000
	Autoimmune neutropenia	1 in 100,000
	Acquired hemophilia	1 in 100,000
	Aplastic Anemia	5 in a million
	Autoimmune lymphoproliferative syndrome	< 1 in a million
	Evans syndrome	< 1 in a million
OPHTHALMOLOGY — EYE	Cogan's syndrome	Rare
	Sympathetic ophthalmia	1 in 10,000
	HLA-B27-associated acute anterior uveitis	1 in 10,000
	Autoimmune-related retinopathy and optic neuritis	Rare
NEPHROLOGY — KIDNEY	Goodpasture's disease	1 in 10,000
PULMONARY — LUNG	Sarcoidosis	8 in 10,000

Figure 5. A partial list of autoimmune diseases involving different organ systems that are assigned to different departments or divisions (or multiple divisions) within the medical field.

Autoimmune diseases should exist in a separate institute or center with hematopoietic stem cell transplantation and other immune cellular therapies for autoimmune diseases as a separate division(s) within that autoimmune institute. Autoimmune diseases should have their own board certification and inclusive training and licensing. However, this would require changing the traditional organizational structure that has arisen within medicine.

The current organization of autoimmune diseases and HSCT for autoimmune diseases suffers from an outdated and arbitrary but worldwide anachronism. HSCT is a new and successful paradigm stuck in the anachronism of medical history and territorial fiefdoms.

Eyes Wide Closed

One opaque hindrance to HSCT is very difficult to self-diagnose: rigid training. The speaker for my medical school graduation class stroked our egos and confidence by complimenting us on our individual accomplishments and the threshold we had achieved by graduating. But then he said something seemingly paradoxical: "Half of the material you were taught is wrong, but no one knows which half it is."

You must start somewhere, and there is so much information to get your arms around that you begin with memorization. But the unintended consequence is that old "facts" become blinders over your eyes. New ideas often come from minds not indoctrinated within a field's memorized dogma. Louis Leakey selected Jane Goodall to study chimpanzees. She had no degree or background in primatology. She was selected for her passion and uncontaminated open mind. Goodall became the first to document human behavior in wild chimpanzees, including the establishment of hunting bands to kill and eat meat and war parties to kill neighboring chimpanzee tribes. It often takes someone not indoctrinated within a field to bring about a paradigm shift.

After my clinical residency and before my clinical fellowship, I had spent seven years in a molecular biology laboratory at the NIH. Late one night, I happened to say hello to a laboratory chief who was sitting behind his desk in another lab at the NIH. Surprisingly, he invited me in for a chat and a cup of fresh coffee that he was brewing. Most people have morning coffee. He was having coffee to fuel himself for a long night of experiments. He was a distinguished laboratory chief and seemed close to retirement. Most people of his age and level of accomplishments had underlings do the experiments, but he knew that the devil is in the details, so he still at times did the hands-on work himself.

It was the only time I spoke with him, but that conversation has stuck with me. He was part of the team that discovered part of the code of life called transfer RNA (tRNA), part of the holy grail of understanding how genes are converted (translated) into proteins. He kept in his lab freezer a piece of the original tRNA from those experiments. Why would he do that? That night this seasoned researcher shared his secret with me: "Research is the art of *re*-searching, of repeating the research." It is repeating the search at another time with different eyes. When you repeat a search, you need to go back to the original source. In fact, that is what I eventually did with stem cell transplantation for autoimmune diseases. I repeated the research performed on aplastic anemia in the 1960s but in different autoimmune diseases, such as multiple sclerosis.

Memory is an evolutionary advance. If early in life you touch something that burns, you remember and avoid it in the future. Memory allows us to learn from past experiences in order to adapt and modify our future actions and relationships. The exact biological mechanisms behind memory are unknown, but neurons that are excited together tend to remain within the same activation circuit. Memory likely involves the production and/or modification of proteins. These proteins likely encode certain fixed responses and patterns of response that do not require production or modification of new proteins when reexposed to that sensory stimulus.

For the neurons involved, once a circuit is encoded, erasing it by dissembling proteins, rerouting new neural circuits, and generating new neural proteins would require considerable cellular effort, likely in the currency of cellular energy—i.e., generation of ATP (adenosine triphosphate). Since nature does not waste energy, it often has no driving reason to erase and reestablish new cognitive circuits. As Pablo Picasso once said, "Every act of creation is also an act of destruction."

The neurophysiology involved in learning, including academic university learning, offers a tremendous survival advantage, but it is also likely that memory is the neurophysiology mechanism behind bias and prejudice. Memory and bias are two sides of the same coin. It takes considerable effort and energy to reestablish cognitive plasticity, and thus new ideas and approaches that come from outside the field are often initially rejected by the established "elites" within a field.

The journal *Nature* is perhaps the most prestigious scientific journal in the world. All people in science, academia, or even in medicine aspire to publish in *Nature* (though *Nature* is not a clinical medical journal, per se). A writer for *Nature* approached me during a meeting at the Vatican in Rome. She congratulated me on my talk, then said she was writing an article and wanted to speak with me. I said "sure." She never returned for a conversation. I never saw or heard from her again until I read her article in *Nature* about the meeting. It was titled "Smoke and Mirrors," and it chastised the "scientifically naïve Vatican" for supporting adult stem cell treatments and ignoring the "ethical implications of false hope."[3]

I was taught that science is open to different thoughts and starts with the null hypothesis: that is, you need to prove that you yourself are wrong. Indeed, that is why I performed randomized trials. I wrote a response to *Nature*, but *Nature* declined, saying they would not publish further responses to the "Smoke and Mirrors" article. This refusal to publish a refuting viewpoint is the antithesis of science.

I am in no way defending any religion, per se. I wrote a response to defend science itself. Because *Nature* declined to publish further responses, and because my response to *Nature's* "Smoke and Mirrors" highlights the entrenched and fixed mindset that may cause one's eyes to be wide closed, my response to "Smoke and Mirrors" follows.

Response to "Smoke and Mirrors"

The Nature *editorial titled "Smoke and Mirrors" on the Second International Vatican Adult Stem Cell meeting held on the 11–13th of April in Vatican City was ironically itself a collection of smoke and mirror appeals to emotion and prejudice.*

The first smoke and mirror is that the author spent a significant portion of the editorial on a recent Italian parliamentary decision to overturn a case on stem cell treatment for children that had been stopped by regulators against the parents' and physicians' wishes. The Italian case alluded to in the editorial was, to our knowledge, not mentioned at the Vatican conference, and to our knowledge, the importance of proper regulatory oversight was never questioned at the Vatican meeting.

No reasonable person doubts the importance of regulations and guidelines, but it should be equally obvious that regulations need to be balanced, realistic, and practical. As Winston Churchill said: "If you have 10,000 regulations, you destroy all respect for the law." To which we may add that if you have 10,000 pages of medical regulations, you destroy all respect for patient care. This is because the devil is in the details, and these details arise daily, hourly, even continuously, between patients, their families, disease, treatment, and their doctors. Complications that cannot be foreseen by a distant and lumbering bureaucracy that is not moved by or intimately aware of everyone's circumstances.

The editorial's language of smoke and mirrors is evident in the selection of prejudicial and emotional phrases. The author stated that it is wrong to "exploit the disabled and terminally ill." No reasonable person would disagree with such a comment, but it does not apply to the Vatican conference. In fact, it is appropriate and not unusual for patients and patient advocacy groups to be involved in meetings to educate people and advocate for new and better therapies for their diseases. Does this author similarly cite and condemn AIDS activists for their role in advancing HIV treatments? The author states that the Vatican is "naïve," but a less sensational and more accurate description of the Vatican's position is altruism. The Vatican has no financial or academic gain in terms of publications or, for that matter, media admiration from holding a stem cell meeting.

The author states that the meeting was "shamelessly choreographed and stem cell companies and scientists who spoke at the meeting were desperate to hawk a message." This generalization denigrates all speakers at the Vatican conference, including a Nobel laureate for his work on cellular reprogramming to an embryonic-like state, as well as other university stem cell researchers and speakers who are not, to our knowledge, affiliated with or seeking affiliation with companies marketing adult stem cells. Perhaps as the smoke and mirrors are removed, it could be said that the Nature *editorial was itself shamelessly choreographed to hawk a message.*

There is no smoke and mirrors in the Vatican ethical position on embryonic stem cells (ESC), and this may explain the editorial's underlying antipathy for anything associated with the Vatican. The editorial, in its antipathy toward the Vatican, minimized adult stem cell research and in so doing appears guilty itself of the smoke and mirror argument of minimizing the promise of one type of stem cell in order to promote another type. In reality, all types of stem cells currently have real potential and real limitations.

It is the role of science to question and re-question assumptions and beliefs. It is not the role of science to intimidate, bully, or vilify.

Appropriate editorial didactic questions for academic discussion should have been: 1) Is the Vatican, which opposes embryonic stem cell work but allowed free discussion of embryonic stem cell research, a proper venue for a stem cell meeting? 2) What is the appropriate role for a company or companies in such meetings, as companies are normally involved in many medical professional meetings?

No person or institution should have their freedom of speech, ethical concerns, or ideas censored or be made to fear retaliation, especially from a scientific journal as prestigious as Nature. On the other hand, there are historical concerns why religion, business, and science require transparency and some level of separation. Unfortunately, the Nature *editorial missed this important opportunity and instead condescended into the stereotypical demagoguery that it was condemning.*

The word education *arises from a Latin root, and in Portuguese, perhaps the most Latin of the Romance languages, the word* educado *means "to be polite." Under stress we all are human with normal emotional responses, but an educated person when having time to reflect and write should attempt to be polite, and that role should be exemplified in the publications of any prestigious science journal. As speakers at the Vatican conference and as researchers who work with both embryonic and adult stem cells, we believe a more polite editorial on the Vatican conference would have been in the best interest of science, society, and patients. Within the limits of its ethical principles, a more accurate description of the Vatican conference would have been: "Open discussion, a first step toward a detente in the stem cell debate?"*

Financial Toxicity

Physicians are not only removed from responsibility in controlling medical costs, but in practice, the opposite scenario often occurs. Excessive revenue collection is encouraged, with an end-of-year salary bonus for higher billing (called RVUs). There is no incentive for being cost-effective. Physicians are not generally taught or educated to think in terms of a patient's cost, least of all cost-effectiveness of a treatment.

In medical publications, physicians are not required to publish quality of life (although that is starting to change) nor costs or comparative costs of treatment. These are not end points required for general medical acceptance or for patient care. Major medical publications omit such information without criticism or second thought. Consequently, most physicians are not consciously aware in their daily practice of how damaging medical costs are for patients or societies that must pay the bill. Patients with exceptional insurance may also be unaware of this until they lose their job and thus, also their medical benefits.

I am not suggesting that cost considerations supersede what is best for the patient that would be an overreach in the wrong direction. Rather, because the patient must be the priority, the cost-effectiveness of treatment (cost versus benefit) needs to be understood. As reported in the multiple sclerosis and chronic inflammatory demyelinating polyradiculoneuropathy disease chapters, it is more cost-effective to convert (using nonmyeloablative HSCT) a chronic autoimmune disease into a one-time reversible illness than to continue following current standards of chronic care. Yet this has not resonated within each disease's subspecialty field. This problem is not unique to HSCT.

As an example, the drug rituximab (Rituxan) that is a protein (monoclonal antibody) directed against B lymphocytes (a type of immune cell) was being used off-label by neurologists for multiple sclerosis. Because the patent on rituximab had expired, and because it had become less expensive, no drug company wanted to study it for its use against multiple sclerosis, despite its published effectiveness. Instead, a pharmaceutical company patented a similar but slightly different anti-B cell monoclonal antibody called Ocrevus (ocrelizumab). When the FDA awarded Ocrevus a license for multiple sclerosis, neurologists stopped using the cheaper and effective patent-expired rituximab and began using the much more expensive patented Ocrevus, that often costs $40,000 per infusion. Why is this? There is a general bias toward drugs with an FDA-licensed indication, which means they have an enforceable nonexpired patent, a market monopoly, and are expensive; otherwise, nobody would perform the expensive study needed to obtain the FDA license. It is a Catch-22 for which the patient pays.

There has been no randomized trial comparing rituximab to Ocrevus in patients with multiple sclerosis, nor in the current environment will there be one. It is highly likely that they would be equally effective, but rituximab would be much cheaper. There is no incentive to compare a new FDA-approved drug to the best non-patented (i.e. patent expired) drug or combination of nonpatented drugs. This problem is not unique for the drug rituximab, nor is it unique to the neurology community. In my prior life as a hematologist/oncologist, I noticed the same problem in oncology (cancer), and in the field of transplant, NIAID advocates for the significantly more expensive myeloablative regimens. Failure to consider the most cost-effective approach is a widespread and endemic problem that allows medical costs to far exceed the rate of inflation.

The system should be tweaked to (a) make physicians aware of medical costs and engage them in cost containment, and (b) in order to do this, protect physicians as independent professionals. What training or policies could be implemented to help accomplish this tweaking?

On a local training and educational level, a physician's medical training and Hippocratic oath should include protecting not just the patient's medical health but also their financial health. Medical and psychological health suffer when toxic costs deprive a patient of financial security. In order to do this, current labyrinthine medical billing codes need to be simplified, and physicians need to be trained in the costs of treatments and their relative benefits in quality of life.

On the state level, a few states have enacted laws that prevent hospitals from hiring physicians as employees. When hospitals own physician practices, it circumvents and legalizes self-referral that would otherwise be a violation of the Stark law against nepotistic practices.[4] A lawyer cannot adequately represent a client if the lawyer is an employee of the prosecuting district attorney or presiding judge in the client's case. To avoid conflict of interest, including financial conflicts between the institution and patient, physicians must be knowledgeable about cost-effectiveness and able to represent patients in a hospital or institution without being conflicted as an employee.

On the national level, advocating for randomized trials to include both quality of life and cost-effectiveness analysis are concepts that may provide checks and balances on toxic medical costs. Medicine is a profession, but whether managed by the government or private sector, healthcare is a business. It is an anachronism to exclude patients and bedside physicians from involvement in and being rewarded for controlling short-term and long-term healthcare costs.

Perhaps the system is too large and self-invested for these modest tweaks to be made possible. On the other hand, the system exists for patients, and from many patients' perspectives, the current system is failing. Medicine and the business of medicine is so complex that it is hard to know how to implement constructive change. Perhaps as a society of individuals, we could start by agreeing to the guiding principle of these 4As: Affordable, Advanced, Accountable, and All-inclusive.[5] A method to establish equilibrium in these competing principles is to implement checks and balances. An independent (nonemployee) physician schooled and allowed to represent the best interests of their patients both financially and medically would act as a brake on runaway medical expenses.

Conclusion

When I was young, my youthful optimism was shaken by the Fyodor Dostoevsky novel *Crime and Punishment* in which no matter what the characters did, human suffering was inevitable and inescapable. Per-haps, as these stories tell, we are not trapped. Human suffering is not inescapable. An idea can change reality. You have one life so follow your instincts." As Fyodor Dostoevsky wrote: "To go wrong in one's own way is better than to go right in someone else's."

Changing a chronic autoimmune disease into an illness that can be reversed with a one-time treatment could not have been accom-plished without academic independence and freedom. Nor could it have been accomplished without the trust and faith of my patients and their families or without the good will of the many people who helped me. For those patients and people who could not be included in this book due to word limit constraints, you are just as much a hero or heroine. Thank you! You have taught me and this world so much!

As the Dalai Lama said: "Grapes must be crushed to make wine. Diamonds form under pressure. Olives are pressed to release oil. Seeds grow in darkness. Whenever you feel crushed, under pressure, pressed, or in darkness, you're in a powerful place of transformation."

NOTES

For more references, go to:

https://astemcelljourney.com/medical-publications/

Chapter 3: Introduction to HSCT for Autoimmune Diseases

1. Richard K. Burt, Dominique Farge, Milton A. Ruiz, Riccardo Sac-cardi, John A. Snowden, *Hematopoietic Stem Cell Transplantation and Cellular Therapies for Autoimmune Diseases* (Baton Rouge: CRC Press, 2021), https://www.routledge.com/Hematopoietic-Stem-Cell-Transplantation-and-Cellular-Therapies-for-Autoimmune/Burt-Farge-Ruiz-Saccardi-Snowden/p/book/9781138558557.
2. National Institute of Allergy and Infectious Diseases (NIH), https://www.niaid.nih.gov.

Chapter 4: Multiple Sclerosis (MS)

1. "The Nobel Prize in Physiology or Medicine 1990," The Nobel Prize, https://www.nobelprize.org/prizes/medicine/1990/summary/.
2. Burt RK et al., "Effects of Disease Stage on Clinical Outcome After Syngeneic Bone Marrow Transplantation for Relapsing Experimental Autoimmune Encephalomyelitis (EAE)," *Blood* 1998 91: 2609–261.
3. Burt RK et al., "Hematopoietic Stem Cell Transplantation for Progressive Multiple Sclerosis: Failure of a Total Body Irradiation–Based Conditioning Regimen to Prevent Disease Progression in Patients with High Disability Scores," *Blood* 2003 Oct; 102(7):2373–8.
4. Mike V et al., "Incidence of Second Malignant Neoplasms in Children: Results of an International Study," *The Lancet* 1982; I: 1326–31.

5. Weiner et al., "Treatment of Multiple Sclerosis with Cyclophospha-mide: Critical Review of Clinical and Immunologic Effects," *Multiple Sclerosis Journal* April 1, 2002.

6. Burt RK et al., "Autologous Nonmyeloablative Hematopoietic Stem Cell Transplantation in Relapsing-Remitting Multiple Sclerosis: A Phase I/II Study," *Lancet Neurology* 2009; 8: 244–53.

7. At the Limits, https://www.atthelimits.org.

8. Baker D, et al., "Interpreting Lymphocyte Reconstitution Data from the Pivotal Phase 3 Trials of Alemtuzumab," *JAMA Neurology* 2017; 74 :961–969.

9. DHCS, https://www.dhcs.ca.gov/services/ccs/Pages/default.aspx.

10. Burt RK et al., "Association of Nonmyeloablative Hematopoi-etic Stem Cell Transplantation with Neurological Disability in Patients with Relapsing-Remitting Multiple Sclerosis," *JAMA* 2015; 313(3):275–284.

11. Hauser SL, "Hematopoietic Stem Cell transplantation for MS: Extra-ordinary Evidence Still Needed," *JAMA* 2015; Jan 20; 313(3):251–2.

12. Burt RK et al., "Health Economics and Patient Outcomes of Hema-topoietic Stem Cell Transplantation Versus Disease-Modifying Therapies for Relapsing-Remitting Multiple Sclerosis in the United States of America," *Multiple Sclerosis and Related Disorders* 45 (2020) 102404.

13. Healy BC, Engler D, Glanz B, Musallam A, Chitnis T, "Assessment of Definitions of Sustained Disease Progression in Relapsing-Remitting Multiple Sclerosis," *Mult Scler Int.* 2013; 2013:189624.

14. Hays RD, Woolley JM, "The Concept of Clinically Meaningful Dif-ference in Health-Related Quality-of-Life Research," *Pharmacoeco-nomics* 2000, Nov, Vol 18 (5): 419–423.

15. Burt et al., "Effect of Nonmyeloablative Hematopoietic Stem Cell Transplantation vs Continued Disease-Modifying Ther-apy on Disease Progression in Patients With Relapsing-Remitting Multiple Sclerosis—A Randomized Clinical Trial," *JAMA* 2019; 321(2):165–174.

16. Hartung DM, Bourdette DN, Ahmed SM, Whitham RH, "The Cost of Multiple Sclerosis Drugs in the US and the Pharmaceutical Indus-try: Too Big to Fail?" *Neurology* 2015;84(21):2185–2192.

17. Hartung DM. Johnston KA, Geddes J, Bourdette DN, "Effect of Generic Glatiramer Acetate on Spending and Use of Drugs for Multiple Sclerosis," *Neurology*. 2020;00:1–8.

18. Hartung DM. Johnston KA, Geddes J, Bourdette DN, "Effect of Generic Glatiramer Acetate," 1–8.

19. Mult Scler, "Pilot Trial of Intravenous Autologous Culture-Expanded Mesenchymal Stem Cell Transplantation in Multiple Sclerosis," *National Library of Medicine* 6 April 2017; 24(4): 501–511, https://www.ncbi.nlm.nih.gov/pmc/articles/PMC5623598/.

20. Auto Immune and Multiple Sclerosis (AIMS), www.aimscharity.org.

21. Burt RK et al., "Real-World Application of Autologous Hematopoietic Stem Cell Transplantation in 507 Patients with Multiple Sclerosis," *Journal of Neurology* 24 September 2021.

22. Burt RK et al., "Real-World Application of Autologous."

Chapter 5: Systemic Sclerosis (Scleroderma)

1. "Cyclophosphamide Versus a Placebo in Scleroderma Lung Disease," *NEJM* 2006;354:2655–66.

2. "Effects of 1-Year Treatment with Cyclophosphamide on Outcomes at 2 Years in Scleroderma Lung Disease," *Am J Respir Crit Care Med* 2007;176:1026–34.

3. Burt RK, et al., "Autologous Nonmyeloablative Hematopoietic Stem Cell Transplantation Compared with Pulse Cyclophosphamide Once Per Month for Systemic Sclerosis (ASSIST): An Open-Label, Randomised Phase 2 Trial," *The Lancet* Vol378 - August 6, 2011.

4. Burt RK, et al. "Cardiac Involvement and Treatment-Related Mortality after Nonmyeloablative Hematopoietic Stem Cell Transplantation with Unselected Autologous Peripheral Blood for Patients with Systemic Sclerosis: A Retrospective Analysis," *The Lancet* January 28, 2013.

5. Burt RK, et al. "Cardiac Involvement and Treatment-Related Mortality."

6. Farge D, et al., "Autologous Hematopoietic Stem Cell Transplantation vs Intravenous Pulse Cyclophosphamide in Diffuse Cutaneous Systemic Sclerosis: A Randomized Clinical Trial." *JAMA* 2014; 311 (24): 2490–2498.

7. Burt RK, et al., "Hematopoietic Stem Cell Transplantation for Systemic Sclerosis: If You Are Confused, Remember: 'It Is a Matter of the Heart,'" *The Journal of Rheumatology* February 2012, 39 (2) 206–209.

8. Burt RK, et al., "Cardiac-Safe Hematopoietic Stem Cell Transplantation for Systemic Sclerosis with Poor Cardiac Function: A Pilot Safety Study that Decreases Neutropenic Interval to 5 Days," *Bone Marrow Transplantation* June 2020.

9. "Myeloablative Autologous Stem Cell Transplantation for Severe Scleroderma," *The New England Journal of Medicine* 2018; 378:35–47.

10. Evans S, "When and How Can Endpoints Be Changed After Initiation of a Randomized Trial," *Plus Clin Trials* 2007 Apr 2(4): e18.

11. Evans S, "When and How Can Endpoints Be Changed," e18.

Chapter 6: Neuromyelitis Optics (NMO)

1. Burt RK et al., "Autologous Nonmyeloablative Hematopoietic Stem Cell Transplantation for Neuromyelitis Optica," *Neurology* October 2019.

2. Traynor AE, Burt RK et al., "Treatment of Severe Systemic Lupus Erythematosus with High-Dose Chemotherapy and Hematopoietic Stem Cell Transplantation: A phase I Study," *The Lancet* 2000;356(9231):701-7.

3. Burt RK et al., "Nonmyeloablative Hematopoietic Stem Cell Transplantation for Systemic Lupus Erythematosus," *JAMA* 2006;295(5):527-35.

4. Greco R et al., "Allogeneic Hematopoietic Stem Cell Transplantation for Neuromyelitis Optics," *Ann Neurology* 2014.

Chapter 7: Chronic Inflammatory Polyneuropathy (CIDP)

1. Burt RK et al., "Hematopoietic Stem Cell Transplantation for Chronic Inflammatory Demyelinating Polyradiculoneuropathy," *Journal of Neurology* 2020.

2. Burt RK et al., "The Cost-Effectiveness of Immunoglobulin vs. Hematopoietic Stem Cell Transplantation for CIDP," *Frontiers in Neurology*, 22 March 2021.

Chapter 8: Crohn's Disease

1. Burt RK et al., "Autologous Nonmyeloablative Hematopoietic Stem Cell Transplantation in Patients with Severe Anti-TNF Refractory Crohn's Disease: Long-Term Follow-Up," *Blood* 2011 Jan.

2. Burt RK et al., "A Pilot Feasibility Study of NonMyeloablative Allogeneic Hematopoietic Stem Cell Transplantation for Refractory Crohn's Disease," *Bone Marrow Transplantation* 2020 May 28.

Chapter 9: Why Can't I Get HSCT?

1. *Hematopoietic Stem Cell Transplantation and Cellular Therapies for Autoimmune Diseases*, Chapters 12, 13, 14. Editors Burt RK, Farge D, Ruiz MA, Saccardi R, Snowden JA. CRC press 2021. Chapters 12, 13, & 14.

2. Aleksandr Solzhenitsyn, *Cancer Ward* (New York: Farrar, Straus & Giroux, 1968), 249.

3. "Smoke and Mirrors," *Nature* 16 April 2013; 496, 269–270 (2013). https://doi.org/10.1038/496269b.

4. Physician Self Referral, Centers for Medicare & Medicaid Services, https://www.cms.gov/Medicare/Fraud-and-Abuse/PhysicianSelf Referral/index.

5. Metzger L. "Is Health Care a Human Right?" In *Hematopoietic Stem Cell Transplantation and Cellular Therapies for Autoimmune Diseases*. Editors Burt RK, Farge D, Ruiz MA, Saccardi R, Snowden JA. CRC Press 2021. Chapter 66.

ABOUT THE AUTHOR

Dr. Richard K. Burt (https://astemcelljourney.com/about/drrichard burt/) is a Fulbright Scholar, Professor of Medicine at Scripps Health Care, tenured retired Professor of Medicine at Northwestern University, and CEO of Genani biotechnology. He endeavored for thirty-five years, first with animal models then with some of the world's first clinical trials, to bring the field of stem cell and cellular therapy to the patients' bedsides. Dr. Burt has published more than 145 mostly first author articles and is the editor of four medical textbooks. He was the first Autoimmune Committee Chairperson for the International Bone Marrow Transplant Registry (IBMTR) and was the principal investigator of a National Institutes of Health (NIH) $10 million dollar multicenter contract to develop stem cell clinical trials for autoimmune diseases. Professor Burt performed America's first hematopoietic stem cell transplant (HSCT) for multiple sclerosis (MS), systemic lupus erythematosus (SLE), Crohn's disease (CD), stiff person syndrome (SPS), and chronic inflammatory demyelinating polyneuropathy (CIDP) and published the world's first randomized clinical stem cell transplantation trials for systemic sclerosis and multiple sclerosis. He has been awarded Leukemia Scholar of America, the Lupus Foundation of America Fidelitas Award, the van Bekkum Award by the European Society for Blood and Marrow Transplantation, the Distinguished Clinical Achievement Award by the Clinical Research Forum, and the European Group for Blood and Marrow

Transplantation Clinical Achievement Award. Dr. Burt was presented in Vatican City, Rome, with the "Keys to the Vatican," was speaker at the Festival of Thinkers in Leadership in Healthcare in the United Arab Emirates, and chaired the biotechnology session at the Baku Azerbaijan International Humanitarian Forum. Dr. Burt was recognized by *Science Illustrated* for accomplishing one of the Top 10 medical breakthroughs for the next ten years and by *Scientific American* as one of the Top 50 individuals, teams, or organizations for improving humanity and outstanding leadership.